LIVING WITH HEPATITIS C

A SURVIVOR'S GUIDE

third edition

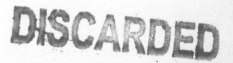

LIVING WITH HEPATITIS C

A SURVIVOR'S GUIDE

third edition

GREGORY T. EVERSON, M.D., F.A.C.P.
HEDY WEINBERG

HATHERLEIGH PRESS

New York

Hatherleigh Press
An affiliate of W.W. Norton & Company
5-22 46th Avenue, Suite 200
Long Island City, NY 11101
1-800-528-2550

DISCLAIMER
This book does not give legal or medical advice.
Always consult your doctor, lawyer, and other professionals.
The names of people who contributed anecdotal material have been changed.

The ideas and suggestions contained in this book are not intended as a substitute for consulting with a physician. All matters regarding your health require medical supervision.

Library of Congress Cataloging-in-Publication Data

TO FOLLOW

ISBN # 1-57826-108-2

All Hatherleigh Press titles are available for special promotions and premiums.
For more information, please contact the manager of our Special Sales department.

Designed by Dede Cummings Designs
Printed in Canada on acid-free paper
10 9 8 7 6

DEDICATION

I wish to thank my family for tolerating my late hours of work, absence from home, and long periods at the computer. Special appreciation and thanks go to my wife, Linda, and sons, Brad and Todd. You truly are my inspiration. I also want to give special recognition to my father, Lloyd K. Everson, who may be one of the oldest students of the computer at age 84, and my mother, Ruth Fursteneau-Everson, who was prematurely plucked from this earth at age 60 by breast cancer. To all my friends and colleagues, I hope you get a chance to read this work and let me know if it is worthy of your readership.

Gregory T. Everson, M.D., F.A.C.P.

To my husband, Michael, my love, a truly good person who stands up for what's right, yet keeps a sense of humor, warmth, and openness. Your support, encouragement, and belief in this book made its creation possible.

And to our children—Ben and Yael, Shira and David, and Adam, who offered help and cheered me on—I'm proud of you, your values, and your strong sense of family.

Hedy Weinberg

We also thank our editor, Heather Ogilvie, for her guidance and valuable suggestions in the preparation of this and previous editions of *Living with Hepatitis C.*

In memory of Fred Kern, Jr., M.D., the authors and the publisher will contribute a portion of the profits from this book to the Kern Research Foundation for the Understanding and Treatment of Gastrointestinal and Liver Diseases to further hepatitis C research.

Kern Foundation
7500 East Dartmouth Avenue, No. 30
Denver, Colorado 80231-4264
Telephone (303) 750-5509
Facsimile (303) 750-4688

The authors would like to thank all those who have contributed to the Kern Foundation to further our research into hepatitis C and liver disease. We especially wish to acknowledge our publisher, Hatherleigh Press, for matching our own contributions of a portion of the profits from *Living with Hepatitis C: A Survivor's Guide* and *My Mom Has Hepatitis C.*

These contributions, supplemented by the Liver Disease Fund at the University of Colorado Medical School, have underwritten the cost of a fully automated high-pressure liquid chromatograph (HPLC). This chromatograph analyzes compounds in blood and saliva that are used to measure liver function. The research goal is to develop tests that more accurately measure liver function and predict a patient's clinical course of disease. These tests are currently being used in HALT C, the NIH-sponsored trial of maintenance interferon to prevent disease progression in patients with chronic hepatitis C.

CONTENTS

PREFACE

L IVING WITH HEPATITIS C: *A Survivor's Guide* grew out of a need I saw at the University of Colorado Health Sciences Center. When the first test for the virus became available around 1990, newly diagnosed patients asked questions but, unfortunately, we physicians had relatively few answers. As the years went by, our knowledge grew, and so did the task of educating the rapidly growing number of people diagnosed with hepatitis C.

To meet the public's need for information about hepatitis C, I began to give lectures specifically targeted to patients and their families. After one lecture, Hedy Weinberg, a hepatitis C patient and writer, approached me and suggested that we turn the lecture series into a guidebook for our patients at the clinic. What began as a simple pamphlet quickly turned into a long-term project that resulted in the publication of the first version of this book in 1997.

As we wrote and rewrote the text, we tried to create a useful guide that would take the patient step-by-step through the process of diagnosis and ongoing care. We tried to anticipate questions, translate medical jargon, and reduce the fear of the unknown. Therefore, we also presented overviews of emotional, financial, and nutritional issues that accompany this chronic illness. We added new chapters dealing with liver cancer, co-infection, and children to our second edition, published in 1999. In these pages you will hear the voices of patients and staff at the University Hospital and the University of Colorado Health Sciences Center who generously contributed their knowledge and experiences and encouraged us to complete the work.

Our third edition (2002) continues to update information and resources while trying to maintain our goal of presenting complex medical terms in language that patients can understand. Readers will find a new chapter that presents and analyzes data from clinical trials of the newest treatment for hepatitis C, pegylated interferons (Chapter 9, Pegylated Interferons, The Emerging Standard-of-Care). We also enlarged the scope of the co-infection chapter to include hepatitis B, as well as HIV/AIDS.

As we prepare each new edition, we note the advances in our knowledge and treatment of hepatitis C. We still have a long way to go to eradicate the virus, but the future looks hopeful.

We continually update this guidebook to help people cope with a disease that affects almost four million Americans. In a short clinical visit, people often keep a "stiff upper lip." But for this book, patients shared their experiences—the funny and hopeful times, as well as the frightening, sad moments. I gained a new appreciation and insight into my patients' lives.

Throughout the book we emphasize the need for thoughtful well-controlled clinical and basic research of hepatitis C. The final chapter speculates on potential breakthroughs in virology, cell biology, and medicine that might lead to a cure of this disease. My own career has been centered on investigation and research. I owe much of my interest to my late mentor, colleague, and friend, Dr. Fred Kern, Jr. The Kern Foundation was established in Dr. Kern's name to foster research into the causes and cures of gastrointestinal and liver disease. Both Hedy and I and Hatherleigh Press contribute a percentage of the proceeds from the sale of this book to the Kern Foundation for the express purpose of advancing research into hepatitis C.

One last word: Although *Living with Hepatitis C: A Survivor's Guide* is a detailed reference guide, it does not replace the advice and care of your physician, nor does it give legal advice. Instead, it is designed solely to educate patients and their families about hepatitis C and how it affects their lives. Consult appropriate specialists and always work closely with your doctor when making medical decisions.

ACKNOWLEDGEMENTS

We appreciate and gratefully acknowledge the hard-working, dedicated members of the Liver Team at the University of Colorado Health Sciences Center, who are always generous with help and support: James Trotter, M.D.; Marcelo Kugelmas, M.D.; Greg Fitz, M.D.; Igal Kam, M.D., Chief of Division of Transplant Surgery; Michael Wachs, M.D.; Thomas Bak, M.D.; Susan Mandell, M.D.; Thomas Beresford, M.D.; Barbara Fey, R.N., M.S.N., Hepatology Nurse; Cathy Ray, R.N., B.S.N., M.A., Hepatology Nurse; Jim Epp, R.N., B.S.N., Hepatology Nurse; Megan Dyer, Lori Carrillo, Ariana Wallack, Administrative Assistants; Chris Tomasi, C.M.A., Medical Assistant; Donna Cornelisse, C.M.A., Medical Technologist; Dawn Schmidt, Medical Assistant; Jennifer DeSanto, R.N., Research Coordinator; Melissa Douglass, R.N., B.S.N., Research Coordinator; Carol McKinley, R.N., Research Coordinator; Radene Showalter, Laboratory Researcher; Sue Sellissen, P.R.A.; Shannon Lauritski; Tracy Steinberg, R.N., M.S., C.C.T.C.; Tim Brackett, R.N.; Mary McClure, R.N.; Michael Talamantes, M.S.S.W., L.C.S.W.

Also from the University of Colorado Health Sciences Center, we thank Robert M. House, M.D., Associate Professor, Director, Residency Training, Department of Psychiatry; Patrick M. Klem, PharmD., B.C.P.S.; Hannis W. Thompson, M.D., Associate Medical Director, Bonfils Blood Center, Director of Transfusion Medicine, University of Colorado Medical School; Steven C. Johnson, M.D., Associate Professor of Medicine, Director of the University Hospital HIV/AIDS Clinical Program; Fabi Imo, Coordinator, Transplant Financial Services; Patty Polski, M.B.A., Manager, Registration and Financial Services; Rev. Julie Swaney, University Hospital Chaplain.

Dr. Everson wishes to further acknowledge the support of the staff at University Hospital and the University of Colorado Health Sciences Center in the care and management of patients with hepatitis C.

From The Children's Hospital in Denver, we thank Michael Narkewicz, M.D., Medical Director of the Pediatric Liver Center and Liver Transplant Program, Associate Professor in Pediatrics at the University of Colorado Medical School, Hewit Andrews Chair in Pediatric Liver Disease, who once again gave generously of his time in reviewing Chapter 13. We also thank Ronald Sokol, M.D., Director of the Pediatric General Clinical Research Center, Professor of Pediatrics at the University of Colorado Medical School, Associate Medical Director of the Pediatric Liver Center; Marjanne Claassen, R.N., M.S., C.N.S., Clinical Nurse Specialist, Pediatric Liver Center Nurse Coordinator; and Nancy Butler Simon, M.S., R.N., C.N.S., C.P.N.P., Advanced Practice Nurse, Pediatric General Clinical Research Center; and the Pediatric Transplant Team, including Fritz Karrer, M.D.

We thank Steve Potter, Public Affairs Specialist, Social Security Administration, Denver, for reviewing our information on Social Security issues; and Meredith Pate-Willig, M.S.W., L.C.S.W., for her invaluable help with the emotional challenges of chronic illness.

Special thanks to Anne Jesse, Executive Director, The Hep C Connection, and to Hep C Connection support group members; the University Hospital Transplant Support Group; Kathy Kinch, Executive Director, Rocky Mountain Chapter of the American Liver Foundation; and all the hepatitis C patients across the country who shared their stories and touched our lives.

FOREWORD

SECOND EDITION (1999)

SINCE THE DISCOVERY of the hepatitis C virus (HCV) in 1989, there has been an explosion of knowledge related to both the virus and the disease it causes. Indeed, over 9,000 medical articles on hepatitis C have been published, and newspapers and magazines have highlighted hepatitis C with increasing frequency. The rapid evolution of knowledge as well as the development of therapies and accurate diagnostic tests have overwhelmed most practicing physicians and their patients.

For individuals who have hepatitis C, the diagnosis often engenders strong emotions, ranging from fear and denial to depression and anger. The reactions of loved ones and close friends, whose support is so crucial for people with hepatitis C, are often constrained by their own fear of contagion and ignorance of the disease. Too often, patients and families find little comfort or confidence in the varied, and often conflicting, information received from their health care providers, friends, newspapers, magazines, or the Internet. There is little wonder that for many people the "C" in hepatitis C has come to stand for "confusion."

Fortunately, Gregory T. Everson, M.D., a noted hepatologist, and Hedy Weinberg, a writer and proactive patient with hepatitis C, responded to this need for information with the first edition of their book *Living with Hepatitis C: A Survivor's Guide* in 1997. The title accurately captured the intent of the book to educate patients and their families about HCV, the disease hepatitis C, the variability and complexity of its natural history and manifestations, the therapeutic options, and the strategies for coping and living with a chronic illness. Combining solid medical information with the perspectives, insights, and experiences of a patient resulted in a particularly appealing and readable book. Sensitivity to patients' perspectives and an emphasis on both scientific and psychosocial aspects of hepatitis C were the right prescription for a diverse audience—patients, families, support groups, nurses, and physicians—who has enthusiastically embraced *Living with Hepatitis C: A Survivor's Guide* as an invaluable resource.

The exponential increase in knowledge about hepatitis C over the past three years clearly mandated a second edition of *Living with Hepatitis C: A Survivor's Guide* to provide a comprehensive update on its natural history, transmission, and advances in therapy. The agreeable synergy of science and humanity that characterized the first edition has been sustained in the second edition with careful revision of the original text and addition of three notable chapters. These new chapters address the significant relationship between hepatitis C and primary liver cancer, the special concerns of patients coinfected with HIV and HCV, and the distinctive issues of children who are infected with HCV. The second edition of *Living with Hepatitis C: A Survivor's Guide* admirably achieves its goals and testifies to the authors' commitment to all the patients, families, nurses, and physicians who are challenged by hepatitis C on a daily basis.

John M. Vierling, M.D., F.A.C.P.
Director of Hepatology and Medical Director
of Liver Transplantation,
Cedars-Sinai Medical Center
Professor of Medicine, UCLA School of Medicine
Chair, Board of Directors
American Liver Foundation

1

WHAT IS HEPATITIS C?

An Introduction

I work for a city agency, and we're required to take annual physicals. This year the doctor asked me to come back for more blood tests. My liver counts were high, he said. That's how I found out I had hepatitis C.

I'm managing. What else can I do? But my wife—she's having a tough time. It's hard to believe, but I had never even heard of hepatitis C before.

Barry

IF YOU'VE JUST BEEN DIAGNOSED with hepatitis C, you have a lot of questions: "What is hepatitis C? How did I acquire the infection? Is there treatment? If I tell them at work, will they fire me?"

Hepatitis C is a viral infection that causes inflammation, injury, and ultimately scarring of the liver. That sounds frightening, but try not to panic. You're not alone. Current estimates indicate that nearly four million people living in the United States have hepatitis C. Although hepatitis C is a serious problem, the infection usually progresses slowly over years or decades. You have time to consider your options.

Take a look at the bottom line. Hepatitis C can be dangerous if it damages your liver to the point of cirrhosis. In fact, 8,000 to 10,000 Americans die each year from liver failure due to hepatitis C—about one in every 400 to 500 patients. Based upon the incidence of hepatitis C in the late 1970s, 1980s, and early 1990s (up to 240,000 new cases each year), projections show that mortality related to hepatitis C will triple by the year 2015.

As you can see from the mortality figures, it's far more likely that you will have to learn to live with the virus until scientists find a cure. That's what this book is about: how to live with and survive hepatitis C.

Hepatitis C is a newly discovered disease. Researchers didn't develop a screening test until 1990—long after the hepatitis C virus had infected millions of people. Before this time, it was impossible to detect hepatitis C in donated blood. As a result, the nation's blood supply became contaminated.

That's what happened to Hedy Weinberg, who's writing this book with me. She was exposed to hepatitis C through an emergency transfusion. Let me introduce you to Hedy, who will tell you her story—a story you'll hear throughout the book, because it's typical of what most people face:

> In 1967, I gave birth to a stillborn baby girl. My uterus ruptured, I almost died, and they gave me five pints of plasma. Twenty-six years later, I found out I had hepatitis C. Looking back, it explains some symptoms I've had over the years: a thyroid condition, a slight blood clotting problem, some depression, and fatigue. The transfusion saved my life—but it gave me hepatitis C.

A Word of Caution: Information in this book does not substitute for the advice of your physician. If you have hepatitis C, you should be under a doctor's care.

In this chapter we'll discuss some basic facts and statistics about hepatitis C, its history and discovery, and information about viruses and other forms of viral hepatitis. Here are the topics we'll cover:

- You Are Not Alone
- A Silent Epidemic
- The Discovery of Hepatitis C

- Understanding Hepatitis C
  - What Is Hepatitis?
  - What Is a Virus?
  - What Is the Hepatitis C Virus (HCV)?
- The Hepatitis Viral Alphabet
  - Hepatitis A
  - Hepatitis B
  - Hepatitis C
  - Hepatitis D
  - Hepatitis E
  - Hepatitis ?F, X, TTV?
  - Hepatitis G
- Hepatitis C: How Close Is a Cure?

You Are Not Alone

If you, or someone you love, has hepatitis C, know that you're not alone. The U.S. Centers for Disease Control and Prevention (CDC) estimate that 1.8 percent of the population, 3.9 million Americans, have been infected; 2.7 million of them are chronically infected. Hepatitis C is also a global problem. The World Health Organization estimates that hepatitis C infects three percent of the world's population: 8.9 million people in Europe and more than 170 million chronic carriers worldwide (see Figure 1A).

It's hard to relate to numbers this big, so let's make the statistics more real. The number of people in the United States currently infected with hepatitis C is triple that of HIV/AIDS, more than five times that of Parkinson's, and more than ten times the number of Americans with multiple sclerosis.

In my state of Colorado, which is quite typical, about 20,000 to 40,000 people have hepatitis C; that's roughly three out of every 350 residents. Although the public doesn't realize it, chronic hepatitis C is the most common reportable infectious disease in the state.

But numbers and statistics don't tell the whole story. When you're diagnosed with hepatitis C, all of a sudden, you feel as alone as you can possibly feel. It's as if an invisible fence has gone up between you and all the other people who don't have hepatitis C. You have an infectious illness; they don't. You're worried about yourself, and you're worried about the people you love. You're angry. Perhaps you even feel ashamed.

FIGURE IA.   GLOBAL PREVALENCE OF HEPATITIS C
WORLD HEALTH ORGANIZATION
(based on published data, update 1999)

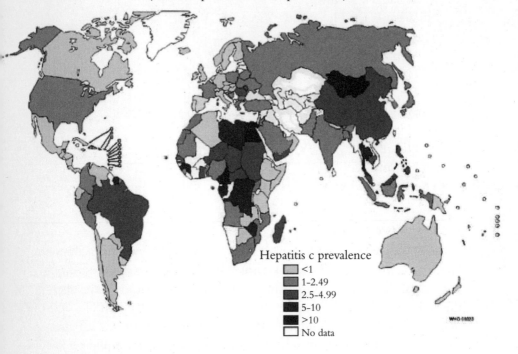

Hepatitis puts a heavy strain on relationships. Mothers and fathers hesitate to cook for their families. Friends who used to hug and kiss you pull away. People don't tell their bosses and co-workers because they fear losing their jobs. Lovers are afraid to touch one another.

> *My wife moved into the other bedroom. The doctor explained that it's okay for us to have sex—that if we're married and we're not sleeping around, there's almost zero risk that she'll get infected.*
>
> *But I don't know. It's like she hears the word "virus," and she freaks out. When I try to hug her, I feel her tense up. It hurts.*
>
> Tony

A healthy dose of facts about hepatitis C helps people deal with their fears. You can touch people; you can cook for them. Tell your family, friends, neighbors, and bosses that to get infected, they'd have to have their skin punctured with contaminated blood. Hepatitis C primarily is a blood-to-blood virus. People get it from transfusions, shared drug needles, tattoos, body piercing, borrowed razors, and so on.

Patients such as hemophiliacs and people on dialysis are at risk because of their exposure to blood and blood products. They make up about 10 percent of the hepatitis C population. Patients with a prior history of blood transfusion account for 20 percent (now, of course, tests screen donated blood for hepatitis C, and the risk of getting hepatitis C from a transfusion is exceedingly low); intravenous drug users represent 20 to 50 percent of cases; and 20 to 40 percent don't know how they came into contact with contaminated blood.

A Silent Epidemic

Hepatitis C is called the silent epidemic because you can have the virus and not know it. It's unusual to have severe symptoms until the end-stages of liver disease—a process that, if it occurs, may take decades. So it's hard for people to believe they're infected. Here's Hedy:

> In December of 1992, I went to my family doctor for a regular checkup. I didn't feel sick, just tired, but that's not unusual for me because I have a thyroid condition. Blood tests showed my liver enzymes were a little above normal. I agreed to stay off alcohol and repeat the tests every month for three months. No change. A specialist ordered more tests and a liver biopsy.
>
> My family doctor called with the results: "Inactive hepatitis C—the best outcome we could hope for." The next day, he phoned again. "There's been a mistake," he said in a sad, tentative voice. "The pathologist reread your slide, and it's mild chronic active hepatitis C."
>
> My stomach clenched. I felt a cold rush of fear, even though I didn't know what hepatitis C was or what to expect.

Hepatitis C usually progresses slowly, with peaks and valleys of activity. Although it's a serious illness, it's important to keep perspective. We now believe that hepatitis C becomes chronic in 55 to 85 percent of infected people.

While it's true that one-third of patients with chronic hepatitis C may develop cirrhosis (scarring of the liver), two-thirds may not. One of five people with cirrhosis may also get hepatocellular carcinoma, a form of liver cancer, but four out of five will not. The frustrating problem is that we can't precisely predict outcomes for individual patients.

A time bomb, the virus can lurk in the body for decades, silently injuring your liver and setting the stage for complications from liver disease.

I had a high-detail, difficult job managing a department store, so at first I thought it was too much stress. I felt foggy, confused. I forgot appointments, couldn't concentrate on the paperwork. Finally, I called a doctor. Maybe I was cracking up. I figured he'd give me an anti-depressant.

Two days before my appointment, my eyes turned yellow, my stomach was out to here, and I itched all over. The diagnosis? Cirrhosis, end-stage liver disease caused by hepatitis C. My life narrowed down to two choices: die or get on a waiting list for a liver transplant.

Jim

We need to get the word out that hepatitis C is a major public health problem. Many people have no idea they're carrying the virus, but it's the most prevalent form of chronic hepatitis in the United States, accounting for 20 to 25 percent of all hepatitis cases. When did this silent epidemic begin?

The Discovery of Hepatitis C

In the 1970s, researchers developed blood tests to identify the viruses that cause hepatitis A and B. However, it became apparent that many blood samples responsible for cases of post-transfusion hepatitis tested negative for A and B. For lack of a better term, scientists called this virus non-A, non-B hepatitis.

Then, in the 1980s—breakthrough! After many years of work, investigators under the direction of Daniel W. Bradley and Michael Houghton at the CDC and Chiron Corporation finally identified the virus in non-A, non-B infected blood. They used specialized genetic chemistry to identify the virus, and with this discovery, they were able to give it a name: hepatitis C.

In 1990 the first test for the hepatitis C virus (HCV) became commercially available. Routine physical examinations and blood bank screens uncovered an explosion of cases.

> *In my mail yesterday was a letter from the blood bank. They had refused my blood because it showed up positive for hepatitis C. What a shock! I couldn't believe it. I've never been sick a day in my life. What is hepatitis C?*
>
> *Tom*

Understanding Hepatitis C

To understand hepatitis C, it helps to define three terms:
- hepatitis
- virus
- hepatitis C virus or HCV

What Is Hepatitis? Hepatitis simply means inflammation of the liver. Many injurious agents can cause hepatitis, including alcohol, medications, drugs, toxins, or viruses.

Unfortunately, the public hears so many stories of celebrities who injured their livers with substance abuse that they tend to lump all forms of liver disease together. As anyone with hepatitis C can tell you, it's not uncommon (although extremely unfair) to be labeled an alcoholic, even if you've never taken a drink.

> *When I finally tell someone I have hepatitis C, the atmosphere changes. I've had people give me this airbrush handshake because they don't want to touch me. Or they'll say, "Isn't that what that baseball star had? Didn't he drink himself to death?" Suddenly, there's this invisible wall.*
>
> *Sara*

During the past 30 years, scientists have discovered hepatitis viruses A through G. Each virus has its own ways of infecting people, but it's hard for the public to see the differences.

> *It's an awkward moment when you let friends know you have this disease. They don't know what to say, and most of what they know about viruses has to do with AIDS, so you get a lot of weird stares and silences. You can see the stereotypes running through their heads. I'm so tired of explaining that the virus is almost never passed sexually, that it's a blood-to-blood thing.*
>
> *Bob*

What Is a Virus? The name virus evokes fear in people, fear of the unknown, the invisible. Viruses are not visible to the human eye or by standard microscopy; you need an electron microscope to see them. Despite their small size, viruses carry genetic material with enough punch to injure our organs and bodies and even cause death.

Viruses are as old as humankind—possibly older. Archeologists have unearthed an Egyptian mummy that bears pockmarks, evidence of the smallpox virus thousands of years ago. Among other diseases, viruses cause polio, mononucleosis, rabies, herpes, yellow fever, influenza, measles, rubella, chickenpox, mumps, the common cold—and new plagues, such as Ebola and AIDS.

"A virus," said Nobel Laureate Sir Peter Medawar, "is a piece of bad news wrapped in protein."[1] And that about sums it up. A virus contains a center of nucleic acid (the viral genes) surrounded by a protein coat.

When a virus's coat attaches to a cell in the body, the virus's genes enter the cell. It orders the cell to stop its own work and to make more viruses instead. In time, the virus multiplies to infect other cells.

Alerted to danger, the body's immune system sends out antibodies, special types of proteins, to stick to the invading virus and neutralize it. Viruses, however, are able to change and mutate to evade these antibodies.

Unfortunately, the hepatitis C virus is particularly good at mutating, which makes it difficult for scientists to create a vaccine. It's been hard to hit this moving target.

What Is the Hepatitis C Virus (HCV)? HCV is a single-stranded ribonucleic acid (RNA) virus organized like the RNA of flaviviruses, a family of viruses that produce yellow fever, dengue, and Japanese encephalitis. To complicate the hepatitis C picture even more, at least six distinct genetic strains (or genotypes) of the HCV virus have been identified.

The Hepatitis Viral Alphabet

When you tell someone you have hepatitis C, you usually end up fielding a lot of questions that have to do with other forms of viral hepatitis: "Do you get it from sex? From dirty food?" It helps to know the facts about the hepatitis alphabet—from A to G. Take Hedy's situation:

> For a long time, I didn't talk about hepatitis C except to my husband and kids. When I finally told a couple of good friends, I don't know what I expected—sympathy, horror. I didn't expect my friend to make light of the whole thing. "Maybe you ate in a dirty restaurant," she said. "No big deal. You'll be fine." I explained how hepatitis A spread.
>
> When I told a second friend, she looked so uncomfortable, I knew she thought I had been infected sexually. I finally convinced her that she was thinking of hepatitis B.
>
> Neither understood, and I felt frustrated and annoyed. I don't know why I was so upset. Before I knew I had hepatitis C, I didn't know what the differences among hepatitis viruses were either. It doesn't make sense, but it took me a long time before I felt ready to talk to a friend again.

As you now know, hepatitis means inflammation of the liver. The most common cause of hepatitis is viral. Hepatitis viruses primarily attack the liver, while other viruses (such as the herpes or mononucleosis viruses) injure the liver as part of a generalized infection.

We know at least seven distinct hepatitis viruses, identified by the letters A through G. Blood tests distinguish and diagnose the different forms, but the public tends to lump them all together.

Hepatitis A. Outbreaks of this virus occur because of poor hygiene—a contaminated water supply or, for example, inadequate hand washing in a day-care facility. Hepatitis A, excreted in feces, is the most common cause of food or waterborne epidemic hepatitis. Areas of high prevalence include Mexico, Central America, Sub-Saharan Africa, Southeast Asia, and the Middle East.

People who contract hepatitis A typically develop flu-like symptoms within 10 to 40 days of exposure (the acute stage). They experience low-grade fever, muscle aches, joint aches, headache, malaise, anorexia, and mild abdominal pain. Often, but not always, these symptoms are rapidly followed by jaundice, a yellowing of the whites of the eyes and skin. In the vast majority of cases, the patient recovers completely with lifelong immunity against re-infection.

Hepatitis A never persists after the acute infection, so people don't develop chronic hepatitis, cirrhosis, or liver cancer. Rarely, in approximately one out of 1,000 cases, does the patient have severe acute hepatitis leading to liver failure and urgent need for transplantation.

An effective vaccine that prevents hepatitis A is available. It is currently recommended that patients with chronic hepatitis C receive hepatitis A vaccine.

Hepatitis B. Hepatitis B spreads primarily through blood inoculation: transfusions of blood or blood products, intravenous illicit drug use, hemodialysis, cardiac bypass surgery, or accidental needle-stick. It also spreads readily by sexual contact, both heterosexual and homosexual, close personal contact, and can easily be transmitted from mother to infant at delivery.

Ninety to 95 percent of adults infected with hepatitis B clear the infection and maintain lifelong immunity. Rarely, a patient may develop liver failure from severe acute hepatitis B. The remaining 5 to 10 percent do not clear the virus. They become carriers or develop chronic hepatitis and risk progression to cirrhosis or liver cancer.

Untreated newborns who acquire hepatitis B from their mothers often develop lifelong infection. The good news is that treating the newborn with HBIG (hepatitis B immune globulin) and hepatitis B vaccine immediately after delivery prevents transmission in more than 95 percent of cases.

People with acute hepatitis B have the same symptoms as people with any other form of acute hepatitis. Chronic sufferers may not have symptoms or may complain of chronic fatigue, malaise, poor energy, and episodic jaundice.

Current FDA-approved medical therapies for chronic hepatitis B are interferon-alfa and lamivudine. Other potentially effective antiviral agents under study include ganciclovir, lobucavir, adefovir, dipivoxil, thymosin-alpha1, and famciclovir. Patients who need transplants for severe acute hepatitis seldom, if ever, develop hepatitis B in the transplanted liver. The virus may recur in transplants performed for chronic liver disease, but use of lamivudine and long-term immune globulin therapy after the transplantation reduces that risk.

A highly effective vaccine that prevents hepatitis B is available. It is currently recommended that patients with chronic hepatitis C receive hepatitis B vaccine.

Hepatitis C. Hepatitis C is transmitted by blood, like hepatitis B. However, unlike hepatitis B, it seems to be poorly transmitted by sexual contact and is infrequently passed (6 percent) from an otherwise healthy mother to her newborn.

> *We've been married 15 years. I told my wife—and the doctor told my wife—that she doesn't have hepatitis C after sleeping with me all these years, and that it would be extremely rare to get it from sex.*
>
> *We could use protection if that would help her feel safer. But it's pretty lonely. She doesn't even hug me anymore.*
>
> *Ralph*

Most infected people may not be aware that they had a past episode of acute hepatitis. In general, symptoms of acute hepatitis C are mild and liver enzyme elevations in the blood are modest. Two chronically infected patients may have identical symptoms and liver enzyme tests but very different results from a biopsy—from mild, benign histology (the study of the liver tissue under the microscope) to advanced injury with cirrhosis.

Patients may be candidates for interferon-based therapy; the current, most widely used is the combination of interferon plus ribavirin. Pegylated interferons are emerging as the next standard-of-care. Other agents under current and future investigation or development include thymosin-alpha-1, ribozymes, histamine analogues, amantidine, inosine monophosphate dehydrogenase inhibitors (IMPDH), antisense oligonucleotides, gamma interferon, and protease and helicase inhibitors.

Today, hepatitis C is the leading indication for liver transplantation. Twenty to 40 percent of patients on liver transplant waiting lists have hepatitis C. The virus recurs in the transplanted liver, and treatment may be necessary.

Hepatitis D. Hepatitis D, or delta hepatitis, is an incomplete virus that requires the presence of hepatitis B in order to complete its life cycle. For this reason, delta is typically found only in patients who have hepatitis B. Most patients with chronic hepatitis B, however, are not co-infected with hepatitis D.

Risk factors are the same as for hepatitis B. Hepatitis B patients co-infected with delta have a greater chance of developing fulminant hepatitis (a sudden, severe attack), more severe chronic active hepatitis, and an increased rate of progression to cirrhosis. The virus does not seem to have a major effect on hepatitis B patients' response to interferon therapy or on their survival or on the recurrence of hepatitis B after a liver transplant.

Hepatitis E. Symptoms are the same as hepatitis A, but cases in the United States appear to be imports from Central America, Mexico, and the Indian subcontinent of Asia. In most instances, patients don't become chronic carriers, and the virus is not associated with hepatocellular cancer.

Currently no vaccine or specific medical therapy exists. If acquired during pregnancy, hepatitis E has been associated with high rates of maternal and fetal mortality. The Centers for Disease Control in Atlanta, GA, offer testing.

Hepatitis ?F, X, TTV? Some patients with viral hepatitis lack evidence for infection with hepatitis A through E. Studies of these patients have uncovered potential new hepatitis viruses. The story is not fully in on these viruses. Early reports have suggested that they may cause sporadic hepatitis, chronic hepatitis, and perhaps progression to liver failure.

Hepatitis G. We're learning more about this newly discovered virus, which is transmitted in the same way as hepatitis C. Hepatitis C and hepatitis G are in the same family of viruses, and hepatitis G is comprised of at least four main subtypes. But we don't know whether hepatitis G causes clinically significant liver disease.

Reports indicate that as many as 20 percent of hepatitis C patients may also be infected with hepatitis G. However, there's no evidence that hepatitis G independently causes chronic progressive hepatitis.

Hepatitis C: How Close Is a Cure?

Viruses are so complex, they can be a frustrating experience for patients who want to know more about them. Here's Hedy's experience:

I'm a p.k.—a preacher's kid—and I'd always been taught that it was good to study and learn and understand. So when I knew I had hepatitis C, I ran to the library.

As a writer, I've done medical research before, but I couldn't make sense out of the numbers and initials and blood types and medical jargon. It was really frustrating. It took a while for me to relax and admit that it was beyond me. It took even longer to realize that part of the problem was that scientists didn't have the answers either.

Researchers have grown the HCV virus in the laboratory and are studying the details of how the virus reproduces. The results could lead to a better understanding of how the virus gains entry to our liver cells and how it reproduces. This knowledge will be instrumental to developing new drugs and therapy to fight hepatitis C.

Recently, several laboratories isolated special enzymes of the hepatitis C virus called helicase and proteases. Researchers anticipate that they will be able to develop specific drugs that will inhibit these enzymes and be highly effective in treating hepatitis C. Similar types of drugs are currently used to treat HIV patients and have been effective in clearing HIV from blood and tissue. The future holds much promise.

Interferon-based treatment has also shown remarkable improvement with progressively increased rates of viral clearance. Remember, the virus was not even identified until 1989. The first interferon trials were for non-A, non-B hepatitis, and only later was it determined that more than 90 percent of the cases were hepatitis C. Initial studies showed that the ALT level normalized in 50 percent of cases, but viral tests were not available. When viral tests became available, we were discouraged to learn that only 10 to 15 percent of patients treated with standard interferon monotherapy cleared the virus.

Combination therapy with ribavirin was the next big step in treatment with interferon. Sustained rates of viral clearance were 38 to 47 percent. Here's Hedy:

I was hesitant to try interferon when I was first diagnosed because I was worried about the side effects, leery of giving myself injections, and concerned about the low rates of success. A second biopsy showed my liver was getting much worse, and that gave me the push I needed to commit to treatment. I started with interferon monotherapy, responded—much to my surprise—then relapsed.

Combination therapy had just become available, and my doctor put me on that right away. I stayed on for a year—a long, hard year—but the results were worth it. Even though I was genotype 1b, I cleared the virus. It's been two years now since I finished treatment, and I'm grateful every day!

Hedy

The newest development is the addition of pegylated interferons. These long-acting forms of interferon in combination with ribavirin result in sustained viral clearance of approximately 55 percent. Studies involving years of following previously treated patients indicate that more than 95 percent of patients who have a sustained viral clearance by six months post-treatment remain free of virus. These data suggest that more than 50 percent of patients treated today may be "cured" of hepatitis C.

As a doctor, I'm excited when a patient conquers and clears the hepatitis C virus. Many patients fail to clear the virus but still have other victories along the way. Any illness, especially a chronic one, tests a person's limits. My hope is that the following chapters will help you learn more about hepatitis C and make you more comfortable with your choices and challenges from day to day.

The beginning of wisdom is to call things by their right names.

Chinese proverb

Reference

1. Peter Radetsky, *The Invisible Invaders: Viruses and the Scientists Who Pursue Them* (Boston: Little Brown and Co., 1994) p. 8.

2

WHEN YOU HAVE
HEPATITIS C

Understanding the Diagnosis:
Blood Tests and Biopsies

For two years I knew there was something wrong. I was tired all the time. In a weird way it was almost a relief when my doctor came up with a diagnosis. Finally, I knew I wasn't crazy or a hypochondriac.

But hepatitis C? My skin wasn't yellow, and I didn't feel that bad. I blurted out the first thing that came into my head: "Did you make a mistake?"

Kevin

"BUT I FEEL FINE!" many of my patients say when I tell them that blood tests show they have hepatitis C. They often follow with, "Are you sure?" All of us, when we hear upsetting news, have the same reaction. A layer of protective denial shelters us from absorbing the news too quickly. We feel almost numb. Then, as our bodies adapt to the increased stress, we start to question. Could there be a mistake?

This chapter answers that question and many others about the testing process for hepatitis C from the time you are diagnosed through the years of ongoing care. It covers the following topics:

• Can Diagnostic Tests Be Wrong?
  ELISA I
  ELISA II, III
  RIBA
  Testing Limits
  HCV-RNA Assays
   1. PCR Assay
   2. Branched-Chain DNA Assay
  Genotyping and Quasispecies
  Liver Imaging Tests
  Ultrasonography (US, Ultrasound)
  Computed Tomography (CT Scan)
  Magnetic Resonance Imaging (MRI)

• Liver Biopsy
  Biopsy Procedure

• Interpreting Biopsy Results

• Liver Blood Tests
  Liver Enzymes
  Bilirubin
  Albumin
  Clotting Factors
  Alpha-Fetoprotein
  Complete Blood Count
  Testing, Testing

Can Diagnostic Tests Be Wrong?

Although current tests for hepatitis C are very good, none are perfectly accurate. Every test has a low rate of both false positives and false negatives. To understand why, you have to learn a little bit about the way these tests work. Most of the tests for hepatitis C measure antibodies that your body produces against the virus. Other tests can actually measure the virus itself (RNA), quantitate levels of the virus, and determine the viral subtype.

When hepatitis C invades the body, your immune system, which is like an army, sends protein "soldiers" into your bloodstream. These proteins are antibodies, and they shape themselves to match molecules (called antigens) on the surface of the virus. The antibodies attach themselves to the hepatitis C virus, and your body's white blood cells then move in to destroy the invader.

The two primary blood tests used to detect hepatitis C, ELISA and RIBA assays, work by reacting to hepatitis C antibodies.

ELISA I. A few months after the discovery of hepatitis C in 1989, ELISA I became available. It detected the antibody for an antigen named C-100. However, ELISA I produced many false-positive results and did not detect the virus in about one-third of cases. If you were diagnosed from 1989 to 1992, and you were never treated or retested, you may want to ask your doctor about repeat testing.

ELISA II, III. In 1993 scientists developed a more sensitive test called ELISA II. The ELISA II assay contains four antigens produced by hepatitis C, so it is more sensitive and specific with fewer false-positive reactions. The ELISA III is the currently used assay and is a further refinement and modification of ELISA II. It was introduced for commercial use in 1996 and has further improved sensitivity and specificity.

Let's go back to the original question, "Can my diagnosis be wrong?" There are still some false-positive reports with current ELISA assays. Nonspecific antibodies may bind to the hepatitis C antigens or react against an enzyme (superoxide dismutase) found in about 3 percent of the normal population. It's a problem of mistaken identity. A positive result with ELISA could be a reaction against the enzyme and not hepatitis C antigens.

The Food and Drug Administration approved a home testing kit for measuring hepatitis C antibodies in 1999. Initial studies suggest that results with this test are similar to standard blood tests.

Resource: The Hepatitis C Check, made by Home Access Health Company of Hoffman Estates, Ill., contains a lancet for obtaining a sample of blood, filter paper, and a mailer. Results are available anonymously by phone through a unique identification number.

RIBA. If you test positive by ELISA, your doctor may decide to confirm the results with RIBA. RIBA is an assay that determines exactly which hepatitis C antigens the antibodies in your blood are reacting to. If your reaction is only against superoxide dismutase, and not against the hepatitis C antigens, you don't have hepatitis C. If you react against two or more hepatitis C antigens, you do have hepatitis C. If you react against only one antigen, then you may or may not have hepatitis C. RNA tests can sort out this diagnostic dilemma.

Testing Limits. The above diagnostic tests measure your antibody response to the hepatitis C virus. They don't measure the virus itself. Antibodies may stay in your body even after you've cleared the virus. A positive result, therefore, means one of the following:

1. You've got an ongoing infection with hepatitis C.
2. You've been exposed to hepatitis C but you're not currently infected. (Some lucky people apparently do fight off HCV on their own, as many as 15 to 45 percent; others may respond to interferon and clear the virus.)
3. You're an infant who received the antibody from your hepatitis-C-infected mother through the placenta. The transferred antibodies usually clear within six to 12 months, unless the baby also becomes infected.

I found out I had hepatitis C when I donated blood and got a letter from the blood bank. What a shock! I didn't go to a doctor right away because I had recently changed jobs and I was waiting for my new insurance papers to arrive. So I joined a support group to find out what the heck I had.

They were all talking about a test that measured the amount of virus in your blood. After my insurance papers came, I had the test done and it came back negative—zero—nothing. Do I have hepatitis C or not?

Karen

HCV-RNA Assays. Karen tested positive for hepatitis C antibodies. But when she took a test that directly measured the virus in her blood, called the HCV-RNA assay, she tested negative. Does she have hepatitis C or not? To answer the question, you need to know that there are two kinds of assays: (1) PCR (Polymerase Chain Reaction) and (2) Branched-Chain DNA.

1. **PCR Assay.** This method is often used for monitoring people on interferon therapy to see if they are clearing the virus. It is not yet known which of the newly developed PCR assays are the most sensitive or specific. Some labs claim that their assay is so sensitive that it can detect as few as 50 virus particles per milliliter of blood. Modifications, such as Transcription Mediated Amplification (TMA) will make these tests even more sensitive.

2. **Branched-Chain DNA Assay.** Chiron Corporation produced the Branched-Chain DNA method. Although the method is easier to apply to a large number of samples, it is relatively insensitive. It measures HCV-RNA levels only above 200,000 viral particles per milliliter.

Getting back to Karen's case, a PCR quantitative assay can give different results at different times. Sensitivity and reproducibility of PCR assays vary among laboratories, and viral levels in your body may fluctuate. Perhaps Karen had only a small amount of virus in her blood, so small the test cannot detect it. If she is retested for HCV-RNA, the virus might show up. On the other hand, Karen may have been exposed to hepatitis C and cleared it. The positive antibody reflects her immune response to the virus.

Here's Hedy's experience:

> *The first time I had a PCR test, the results were mathematical gobbledygook: 5.5 x 10^6 viral particles per milliliter of blood. What does that mean? Is that high? Low?*
>
> *I wanted to hear that I had a low level of virus. For days, I was quietly depressed. Many months later, I had another PCR. I was prepared to hear I had the same or higher results. To my surprise, the viral count was down, way down. I was glad, but it also made me begin to accept how little control I have over this virus.*

What do the numbers mean? What's high and what's low? Anything less than 2 x 10^6 is low. A number greater than 2 x 10^6 is considered high.

Genotyping and Quasispecies. After you've gone through these tests, you may want to know your genotype (subtype). The hepatitis C virus is really a whole family of viruses with six major subtypes. In the United States, types 1a and 1b account for 70 to 75 percent of cases. Different subtypes are more common elsewhere in the world.

Why is this important? We've learned that the subtypes respond differently to therapy. Subtypes 1a and 1b are relatively resistant to antiviral therapy. By contrast, subtypes 2 and 3 seem to respond better. However, we still can't accurately predict success or failure of therapy in an individual based on the HCV subtype. I've seen patients with all subtypes respond to therapy. Here's Hedy:

> When I learned that my genotype is 1b, I became even more leery of treatment. Other statistics also worked against me. I was older, I'd been infected for more than 30 years, and my latest biopsy was worse.
>
> I felt pretty sorry for myself until my sense of humor kicked in. So what if I wasn't a risk-taker? So what if I wasn't lucky, and the only lottery prize I ever won was an ugly crocheted hat at a charity bazaar? It was way past time to start treatment. I'd do whatever I had to do—and give it my best.
>
> Combination therapy worked for me. Two years later, I'm still in remission.

Another predictor of response to therapy may be the number of quasispecies of hepatitis C circulating in the patient's blood. Because the virus mutates so freely, patients often have multiple copies of the hepatitis C virus that vary genetically. This phenomenon is called quasispecies, meaning that the hepatitis C infection actually exists as a diverse set of hepatitis C RNAs within a given subtype.

Patients with the largest number of quasispecies may have more aggressive liver disease and a higher failure rate when treated with antiviral therapy. Patients who have had hepatitis C infection for longer periods of time are more likely to have a greater number of quasispecies. Currently, there are no commercially available tests to establish the degree of quasispecies within a given patient. These studies have been conducted primarily by research labs.

Liver Imaging Tests. Don't be alarmed if your doctor orders an ultrasound or a CT scan. The tests are non-invasive and give information about your liver.

Ultrasonography (US, Ultrasound). Ultrasonography is a safe and painless way to investigate the size, structure, and the vascular (blood) supply of the liver. It's the preferred radiologic technique for an initial assessment for liver tumors.

FIGURE 2A. CT SCANS OF NORMAL LIVER, CIRRHOTIC LIVER, AND LIVER TUMOR (HEPATOMA)

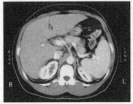
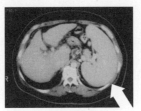
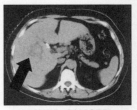

| NONCIRRHOTIC | CIRRHOTIC | LIVER CANCER (HEPATOMA) |

LEGEND 2A: CT scans are specialized radiologic tests that allow one to peer inside the abdomen. The image on the left demonstrates a normal liver and spleen. The middle panel depicts a liver with a knobby irregular surface and an enlarged spleen (⇨) in a cirrhotic patient. The image to the right shows a liver cancer (hepatoma) in the middle of the liver (➡). The patient with the cancer was treated by chemoembolization of the tumor and liver transplantation and is currently alive without evidence of tumor.

Ultrasonic waves penetrate the body tissues and a recording device picks up reflected sound waves that yield an image of the liver. You can compare it to exploring for oil by using seismographic recordings of the earth's formations.

Here's what ultrasound helps find out: liver size and texture and the size of bile ducts and blood vessels. Doppler probes added to ultrasound can detect direction and rates of blood flow in vessels going to and from the liver. Your physician may order ultrasound to pinpoint the liver's location just before a biopsy.

Computed Tomography (CT Scan). Unlike ultrasound, computed tomography (CT scan) uses a highly sophisticated X-ray machine to scan the internal organs with minimal radiation. CT scans are used to confirm the findings of ultrasound and to get a clearer view because, unlike ultrasound, CT scans aren't blocked by air in the bowel. The scans are also more standardized and much less dependent on the expertise of the technician performing the test. CT scans define the size and texture of the liver and can detect an early liver tumor (see Figure 2A).

Magnetic Resonance Imaging (MRI). Unlike ultrasound and CT scans, MRI measures special signals from the body's water molecules. Images are created from these signals. Magnetic resonance imaging is used mainly to diagnose liver cancers.

Liver Biopsy

Just the word "biopsy" strikes fear into people's hearts, but it's an essential part of your treatment. Only a biopsy can give your doctor a true idea of the condition of your liver. You need a biopsy for two reasons:

1. It confirms the diagnosis and rules out other disorders, such as granulomatous liver disease, infections, or biliary tract disorders. Liver biopsy along with ultrasound or a CT scan can be used to pinpoint the site of a lesion and rule out liver cancers.
2. It establishes the stage and degree of activity of hepatitis C. Typically, chronic viral hepatitis passes in sequence from a mild inflammatory stage to fibrosis and, later, cirrhosis. Biopsies may be done over many years to record the progression. Once cirrhosis has developed, there is little reason to continue the biopsies.

Biopsy Procedure. Years ago, liver biopsies were often performed under general anesthesia and required a short hospital stay. Today it's an outpatient procedure that literally takes seconds. In fact, you'll spend most of your time getting ready for the biopsy. However, it is invasive, and you will be asked to sign an informed consent form. It's a good idea to select a doctor who frequently performs this procedure and is very familiar with it. Biopsies may be performed every three to five years.

> I didn't tell my wife I tested positive for hepatitis C; I didn't want to worry her. When my doctor ordered a biopsy and explained what it was, I figured "piece of cake."
>
> I took the afternoon off from work and drove myself to the hospital and back, but we had tickets to a play that evening. I got back home with no time to rest. The play was a bad idea. We had to leave early, and the whole story came tumbling out. That was the end of my macho phase.
>
> Kevin

As you can see from Kevin's story, it's helpful to plan a quiet, restful period after a biopsy. In my experience, most patients' fears come from not knowing what to expect. Here's how the procedure goes:

Your physician examines you carefully to decide exactly where to place the biopsy needle and cleanse the skin with iodine or an antiseptic solution. Then you'll get a local anesthetic, as you do at the dentist's, at the spot where the biopsy needle will be placed. Some doctors also prescribe intravenous benzodiazepine with a narcotic to lessen the anxiety and discomfort.

You'll feel strong pressure when the needle is inserted, but the whole procedure takes only a few seconds for a small core of tissue to be obtained. Then you'll be rolled onto your right side to help control any bleeding from the surface of the liver. You'll stay in the procedure area for two to four hours for observation. If you're stable, with no symptoms, you'll be discharged. Otherwise, you may be admitted to the hospital for observation.

After performing biopsies on hundreds of patients, I've seen very few complications. Reported rates vary from 1 percent to 0.1 percent. If the most common complication occurs, bleeding from the surface of the liver, the patient may require transfusions or even an operation. In rare cases, the biopsy needle may pierce another organ, such as the bowel, gallbladder, kidney, or lung. Death occurs very rarely, in less than one in 1,000 cases.

Interpreting Biopsy Results

Your doctor will tell you the results of your biopsy in terms of histologic stages. Histology means the examination of tissue under the microscope. There are four histologic stages in liver injury due to hepatitis C:

- **Stage I** is characterized by inflammation without the development of any scar tissue.
- **Stage II** features include inflammation with early scarring (fibrosis) in one zone (portal) of the liver.
- **Stage III** shows bridging of the fibrosis between adjacent portal tracts.
- **Stage IV** is cirrhosis (advanced scarring with loss of normal liver architecture).

Histologic stages don't correspond very well to the duration of infection. For example, a patient with slowly progressive disease may maintain an early histologic stage for many years or even decades. Another

FIGURE 2B. HISTOLOGIC STAGES OF HEPATITIS B

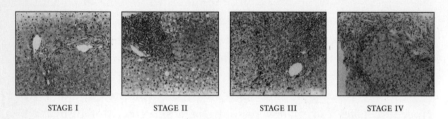

STAGE I   STAGE II   STAGE III   STAGE IV

LEGEND 2B: This figure demonstrates the progressive microscopic changes that may occur in livers infected with viral hepatitis. Stage I shows only mild inflammation in the portal tract; stage II exhibits more inflammation with spread of fibrosis (scar tissue) into adjacent liver cells; stage III implies that fibrosis has spread between portal tracts; stage IV is cirrhosis with formation of nodules.

patient may progress to cirrhosis in less than a decade. The stages of liver damage are distinctive under the microscope (see Figure 2B).

Physicians use certain specific terms when interpreting liver biopsies from patients with hepatitis C. Here's a quick translation:

Stage of Disease	Terminology
Early stage, mild activity (I)	Chronic Persistent Hepatitis C or Mild Chronic Active Hepatitis C
Intermediate stage (II or III)	Chronic Active Hepatitis C with Fibrosis
Advanced stage (IV)	Cirrhosis

Liver Blood Tests

Life with hepatitis C means lots of blood tests to monitor your condition. Have you ever wondered what the numbers really mean? Read the next few pages to review and understand the warning signals of five basic blood tests:

1. enzymes
2. bilirubin
3. albumin

4. clotting factors
5. complete blood count

Doctors frequently test blood in viral hepatitis patients because blood tests warn of changes. The most informative tests "dip" into this bloodstream to measure liver injury (enzymes) or assess liver function (bilirubin, albumin, clotting factors, complete blood count). At first, you may feel intimidated by medical terminology, acronyms, and numbers, but learning about these basic tests will help you understand your doctor's interpretation of results (see Table 2A). Hedy says:

> Who ever heard of this complicated stuff before hepatitis C? At first, I kept track of my liver enzymes religiously, writing each ALT and AST score on a yellow legal pad. I ignored the other numbers on the lab report.
>
> Now I understand that the other function tests let me know how my liver is coping with the infection—like looking into the liver without a microscope. I always ask for a copy of my test results, and I keep my own file. It helps me feel as if I'm doing all I can on my end.

Liver Enzymes. A liver cell produces proteins, called enzymes, that live within the cell or its membranes. In a way, you can think of your liver as a powerful chemical factory; it changes raw materials into the substances your body needs. Enzymes are catalysts that help a liver cell do its job of creating the specific chemical changes that give your body fuel to live. Here are the names of the enzymes you need to remember:

• ALT (SGPT)—alanine aminotransferase
• AST (SGOT)—aspartate aminotransferase
• GGT—gamma-glutamyl transferase
• alkaline phosphatase

By measuring their level in your blood, doctors can monitor ongoing liver injury. Why? Under normal conditions, the level of these enzymes in your bloodstream is relatively low. But when liver cells are injured, destroyed, or die, the cell becomes leaky, and the enzymes escape into the blood that's circulating through the liver. When the cell is injured, liver enzyme levels in the blood rise.

TABLE 2A. NORMAL AND ABNORMAL VALUES
FOR LABORATORY TESTS

Test	Normal Range	Abnormal Range	
		Mild to Moderate	Severe
Liver Enzymes			
AST	< 40 IU/L	40–200	> 200
ALT	< 40 IU/L	40–200	> 200
GGT	< 60 IU/L	60–200	> 200
Alkaline Phosphatase	<112 IU/L	112–300	> 300
Liver Function Tests			
Bilirubin	< 1.2 mg/dl	1.2–2.5	> 2.5
Albumin	3.5–4.5 g/dl	3.0–3.5	< 3.0
Prothrombin Time	< 14 seconds	14–17	> 17
Blood Count			
WBC	> 6000	3000–6000	< 3000
HCT	> 40	35–40	< 35
Platelets	> 150,000	100,000–150,000	< 100,000

KEY:
IU = International Units
l = liter
dl = deciliter
mg = milligrams
AST (SGOT) = aspartate aminotransferase
ALT (SGPT) = alanine aminotransferase
GGT = gamma-glutamyl transferase
WBC = white blood count
HCT = hematocrit (percentage of blood occupied by red blood cells)

Massive liver injury is associated with marked increases in ALT; mild injury may be associated with mild—or even no—increase in ALT. The correlation is strongest at earlier stages of hepatitis C, before the development of cirrhosis. However, once cirrhosis occurs, ALT levels may not be high; therefore, ALT is no longer a good indicator of further liver damage.

What do the numbers mean? Table 2A shows normal and abnormal test values. Blood test patterns relate somewhat to the type of liver injury. Typical hepatitis C patients show increases in ALT and AST but little or no increase in GGT and alkaline phosphatase. Those with cirrhosis or who have an underlying disorder of the biliary tract (the ducts that drain bile from the liver into the intestine) may have modest elevations in GGT and alkaline phosphatase. In some unusual cases of hepatitis C, I have even seen a predominant elevation in GGT.

Patients tend to focus on their ALT and AST counts, but other tests are more important in measuring the health of your liver.

Bilirubin.

After the birth of my second child—a cesarean delivery that required blood transfusions—I learned I was infected with hepatitis C. My AST and ALT counts were only slightly elevated. The most important thing to me was raising my little boys as best I could for as long as I could. I wanted them to know their mother. So I decided to delay treatment and watch my bloodwork every three months.

I made it to my youngest son's ninth birthday when the test pattern changed. "Your bilirubin is up," my doctor said. "It's time to start interferon."

There went the PTA and baking cupcakes—but I did respond to interferon. A good trade.

Jill

When red blood cells complete their life cycle and break down naturally in your body, they produce a yellow pigment that's passed to the liver and excreted into bile. Bile helps your body digest food, but the pigment, which has no digestive function, is called bilirubin. Blood levels of bilirubin tend to fluctuate in patients with hepatitis, although a prolonged persistent elevation in bilirubin usually means severe liver dysfunction and possibly cirrhosis.

Here's why. Most of the time, the body produces as many red blood cells as it breaks down, so you produce a constant amount of bilirubin. However, if your blood cells break down more rapidly (hemolysis) or your liver function becomes impaired, the bilirubin levels in your blood rise.

Your liver has to go to work to take up the excess bilirubin into the liver cell, metabolize it to make it more water-soluble for excretion into bile, and send it through special passages and ducts into the intestine. Microbes in the gut continue to metabolize the bilirubin until you expel it. (Stercobilin, a brown pigment derived from bilirubin, creates the dark brown color of feces.)

When the liver fails to eliminate bilirubin from the blood, the skin and whites of the eyes turn yellow (jaundice), urine darkens, and the color of the bowel movement lightens. In case you've wondered, now you know why your doctor asks you probing questions about the color of your feces.

Albumin. Albumin is another protein synthesized (manufactured) by the liver. Liver cells secrete albumin to maintain the volume of blood in arteries and veins. When albumin levels drop to extremely low levels, fluid may leak out of the blood vessels into the surrounding tissues. This causes swelling, known as edema. Normal albumin levels range between 3.5 to 4.5 grams/deciliter. Usually, edema occurs when levels drop below 2.5 grams/deciliter.

Unlike liver enzyme increases, which occur within hours to days of the liver injury, albumin levels don't fall unless there has been chronic progressive liver injury for at least one month or more. This is because albumin has a long residence time in the plasma; its half-life is approximately 30 days. A decrease in serum albumin, therefore, reflects a slowly progressive, ongoing reduction in the liver's ability to synthesize this protein.

Be aware that there are non-liver reasons for albumin to decrease and your physician will take these into account when interpreting test results. Nonetheless, a significant sustained decrease in serum albumin may mean poor liver function and cirrhosis of the liver. Patients with very low albumin counts may need to be considered for liver transplantation.

Clotting Factors. Remember our comparison of the liver to a chemical factory? The liver also synthesizes many proteins that maintain normal blood clotting. Prothrombin time (PT) is the name of the most common test that measures a combination of blood clotting factors. If your prothrombin time increases, it means your liver isn't creating enough factors, so it takes your blood longer to clot.

Unlike albumin, clotting factors can decrease rapidly—within days, or even hours, of a severe liver injury. In severe cases, clotting disturbances may signal the need for an early transplant. In patients with chronic hepatitis and chronic liver disease, a prolonged prothrombin time can be a warning that the liver is having trouble with its synthetic functions.

Typically, doctors will administer vitamin K, a vitamin essential for normal clotting factors, to determine whether the clotting disorder is reversible. Patients who have persistent, prolonged elevations in prothrombin time that don't respond to vitamin K may need to be considered for liver transplantation.

Alpha-Fetoprotein. This is a protein that regenerative cells or cancer cells secrete into blood. Increased blood levels of alpha-fetoprotein may indicate the development of liver cancer (see Chapter 11).

Complete Blood Count. The complete blood count test can be a detection system for liver scarring. Blood from your spleen flows through your liver via the portal vein. When the liver becomes scarred, it creates resistance to this blood flow (called portal hypertension), and the blood may back up into the spleen. When this happens, the spleen enlarges and traps blood elements, removing them from circulation and lowering blood counts.

Although all components of the blood count may decrease, those most sensitive to this condition are the white blood cell and platelet counts. Patients with portal hypertension from cirrhosis of the liver often have low counts. Similarly, patients may have an enlarged spleen, resulting from severe cirrhotic disease, and may need to be considered for liver transplantation.

Testing, Testing. In the past few years, I've seen the advancement of specific new tests that help monitor your health. But all too often I find that patients feel shut out by the complicated language of test results. Don't worry if you didn't absorb every detail. Use these pages as a reference guide.

Ask for copies of your tests. When you have questions, look up the explanations in these pages. Often, your physician can calm your fears if you voice them. Talk with your doctor.

Knowledge is power.

Francis Bacon

3

WHY ME?
WHAT ABOUT THEM?

How You Got Infected and How to Avoid Infecting Others

When my doctor told me I had hepatitis C, I said, "No way! You've got the wrong blood test. It's got to be some kind of mix-up."

I've never had a transfusion or done drugs. Even when I had my ears pierced, it was with those disposable studs. I mean, I'm a really cautious person. What did I do to deserve this?

Juliana

WHEN YOU'RE DEALING with a serious illness, it's the most human thing in the world to ask, "Why me? What did I do to get hepatitis C?"

The answer is both simple and complex. Most likely you acquired hepatitis C when you came into contact with blood infected with the virus, and it gained entry into your bloodstream.

The complicating factor is that as many as 20 to 40 percent of people with hepatitis C fail to report the way in which they were exposed to infectious blood. And, unlike hepatitis A or B, patients rarely recall a severe initial attack of the disease to mark the time of infection.

How did you get hepatitis C? And how can you avoid giving the virus to others? We'll discuss ways to protect your family and friends. In addition, we'll provide up-to-date summaries of documented ways that hepatitis C is transmitted, including:

- Intravenous Drug Abuse
- Intranasal Use of Cocaine
- Transfusion of Blood or Blood Products
    Surgery or Medical Treatment
    Hemophilia
    Blood Bank Lookback Letters
- Needle-Stick Accidents
- Tattooing and Body Piercing
- Sharing Sharp Instruments
- Birth and Delivery (rare)
- Sexual Transmission (rare)
- Organ Transplantation (rare)
- How Can I Avoid Infecting Others?

Intravenous Drug Abuse

What's the most direct way to get hepatitis C? Inoculate the virus from infected blood into your own bloodstream. That's why one of the most common risk factors is a history of using intravenous illicit drugs. Many drug addicts share needles. They spread hepatitis among themselves and maintain a pool of infected people. Studies suggest that more than 75 percent of current or past users of intravenous drugs may have hepatitis C.

Although heavy drug abusers may be at greatest risk, many people who have hepatitis C report only rare experimentation in the distant past. Unfortunately, the wise decision to stop taking drugs doesn't erase the risk from prior use.

I'm a therapist. People come to me for help with drug abuse. But 20 years ago, when I was a college freshman, I went a little wild. For the

first time I was away from home, and I did some drugs. And yes, I shared
needles once or twice. If only I could go back and change what I did....

Jake

When I question patients about how they got the virus, they usually don't have a clue. I ask them if they've had transfusions or experimented with intravenous drugs. They're shocked. "Can that do it?" they'll say. "It was only once or twice."

When we don't know how the person got hepatitis C, we call it "sporadic" or "community acquired." Some doctors think that most of these cases are due to prior use of intravenous drugs. Patients who are otherwise healthy, employed, and raising their families are stunned to hear they have hepatitis C. They can't believe the diagnosis relates to a past, seemingly insignificant experiment so long ago.

"I don't know how I could get hepatitis C from sharing needles. I was always so careful about cleaning them," patients often say. But to understand how contamination occurs, you have to appreciate how concentrated the virus is in the blood of infected patients.

The average patient with chronic hepatitis C has a blood concentration of the virus of two million particles per milliliter of whole blood. That's equivalent to 2,000 particles of virus in the amount of blood that would sit on the head of a small stickpin. With this concentration it's easy to see that wiping or rinsing a needle with water or salt solutions won't remove all the virus particles. Indeed, a large amount of virus may remain on the needle.

A concentrated solution of hydrogen peroxide will kill or inactivate the virus, and cleaning needles with this solution may reduce the risk of transmission. It won't protect you, however, if cleaning is superficial, such as a quick rinse, or if the internal chamber of the needle is not irrigated and the syringe and all its external and internal parts are not cleansed. Some people rely on others to clean a syringe and don't realize that it's not done thoroughly.

We Americans face a tremendous public health problem from illegal drug use. According to the 1999 National Household Survey on Drug Abuse of Americans age 12 and older, an estimated 6.4 million Americans were currently users of illicit drugs, other than or with marijuana and hashish. An estimated 1.5 million currently used cocaine, and an estimated 200,000 currently used heroin.

On a personal level, the risk factor rises each time you use drugs. If you shoot up once, you may or may not get hepatitis C. But if you shoot up many times, you can almost count on it. The best way to avoid the risk is to avoid illicit intravenous drugs and to teach the next generation to avoid this dangerous behavior.

Intranasal Use of Cocaine

At the time of the NIH Consensus Conference in 1997, researchers thought that 40 percent of patients lacked a known risk factor for acquiring hepatitis C. This led investigators to examine other potential routes of transmission, including snorting cocaine.

Cocaine causes constriction of the blood vessels in the mucous membrane of the nose, leading to disruption of the lining and ulceration. A well-known consequence of chronic cocaine use is necrosis of the nasal septum, leaving a hole in the cartilage that separates the two nostrils. Sharing straws during cocaine use, therefore, can lead to blood-to-blood transmission of hepatitis C. A recent epidemiological study[1] for risk factors for hepatitis C highly correlated hepatitis C with patients who were regular users of cocaine.

Transfusion of Blood or Blood Products

The risk of getting hepatitis C from the transfusion of blood or blood products has been steadily declining since the mid-1980s. Before 1986, there was virtually no screening of blood donors for hepatitis C (then called Non A/Non B), except for sporadic ALT testing. In 1986, blood banks throughout the United States began screening blood donors for hepatitis by measuring ALT (a liver enzyme) and hepatitis B core antibody. Use of these tests by blood banks reduced the risk of acquiring hepatitis C by transfusion one hundred-fold.

Two recent, widely quoted studies (see Table 3A) reported the per unit transfusion risk for the screening procedures. As you can see, scientists developed a test for hepatitis C in 1990 and then improved it in 1992. As a result, the risk of contracting the virus from transfusions went way down.

I'd never been sick a day in my life. Then in 1974, I had a car crash and received multiple blood transfusions.

After the accident, things were never the same. I used to play ball, but heck—it got to where I was always so tired, I could barely go to the games. Forget playing in them.

Terry

TABLE 3A. RISK OF POST–TRANSFUSION HEPATITIS C

Era	Test screening	Cases per 10,000 units transfused
Prior to 1986	None	45
1986–1990	ALT, HBcAb (HIV-Ab, 1985)	19
1990–1991	HCV-Ab, EIA 1	3
1992–1993	HCV-Ab, EIA 2	0.4

You may be wondering if there is currently any risk at all. If a blood donor was recently exposed to hepatitis C, he may be in the "window period" before antibodies form and will therefore test negative. The virus, however, is circulating in his blood and will be passed on to a recipient if the blood is used for transfusion. For this reason, statisticians estimate the risk of infection as extremely low, but there's no such thing as zero risk.

Surgery or Medical Treatment. Certain medical procedures and operations were particularly associated with risk of acquiring hepatitis C due to the large number of transfusions required. These included hemodialysis, coronary artery bypass or heart surgery, lung resection, and major abdominal surgery.

Hemophilia. People with hemophilia lack certain clotting factors in their blood. In the past hemophiliacs were treated with plasma from a large number of donors. The plasma was combined and treated to extract those clotting factors.

Until the mid-1980s, hemophiliacs were at extreme risk for getting hepatitis B and HIV. Therefore, scientists pasteurized the clotting factor for hemophiliacs and this treatment inactivated the hepatitis C virus. When tests for hepatitis C became available in 1990, studies showed that hemophiliacs treated with unpasteurized preparations had an 80 to 90 percent chance of having hepatitis C, while those who received the pasteurized preparation had an extremely low risk, approaching zero percent. Today, current therapy often uses synthesized or genetically engineered clotting products with a zero risk of transmitting hepatitis C.

Resource: For more information, contact the National Hemophilia Foundation at 1-800-424-2634; website: www.hemophilia.org.

Blood Bank Lookback Letters. Today the risk of contracting hepatitis C from blood transfusions is very low because blood banks notify donors who test positive and do not use their blood. Unfortunately, estimates show that contaminated blood transfusions may have infected as many as 300,000 Americans before screening tests were created in 1990 and before highly reliable screening tests were used in mid-1992. Most of these individuals have no knowledge they are infected because they lack symptoms, and therefore, they don't report to physicians. Current estimates suggest that only 10 to 30 percent of patients with hepatitis C have been diagnosed.

The question arose: Should blood banks "look back" and notify recipients of blood from donors who later tested positive for hepatitis C? In March 1998 the Food and Drug Administration (Center for Biologics Evaluation and Research) with the U.S. Department of Health and Human Services issued guidelines for notifying people who may have received infected blood. The guidelines cited recent improvements in the treatment and management of hepatitis C as the motivating reason for the lookback.

Here's how the lookback works. When a donor tests positive, the blood bank must go back ten years to find the people who received blood from this donor (when such records exist) or 12 months prior to the donor's most recent negative blood test. The blood bank notifies the hospital or transfusion service, which must make three attempts to contact the patient's physician. The physician is asked to notify the recipient of the need for hepatitis C testing and counseling.

Unfortunately, it's often difficult to locate at-risk recipients. Many have changed residences and doctors. When donors move from state to state and then turn up hepatitis C positive, previous donations must be traced. Although professionals have long discussed creating a national donor registry, it doesn't yet exist. The Red Cross has a national registry but accounts for only about half of the nation's blood system.

According to Hannis W. Thompson, M.D., Associate Medical Director of the Bonfils Blood Center and Director of Transfusion Medicine at the University of Colorado Medical School, "One infected donor may have given blood 12 times. Each donation may result in three products: red blood cells, fresh frozen plasma, and platelets. That means as many as 36 different people received potentially contaminated blood and must be notified."

Despite all the difficulties, the lookback effort is a positive step. It will help to identify more patients and alert the public to the extent of the hepatitis C epidemic. However, it is my opinion that efforts also should be made to directly notify the at-risk public. If you received blood transfusions prior to 1992, you may be at risk for having hepatitis C today. Consult your physician to see if you should be tested.

Needle-Stick Accidents

Health care workers face an occupational hazard: needle-stick accidents. Because many hospitalized patients and people who frequent emergency rooms have hepatitis, medical personnel run high risks if they accidentally get stuck with an infected needle, which can easily pierce rubber gloves. Here's Hedy:

> I watched the lab tech tie a rubber band around my arm. "I have hepatitis C," I said, noticing that she wore only one glove, so she could probe my skin to check for a 'good' vein. "You might want to put on another glove."
>
> "That's okay," she said, smiling. "I've got hepatitis C, too."

In one study of an inner city emergency room at Johns Hopkins Hospital in Baltimore, MD, 24 percent of 2,523 patients over age 15 were infected with at least one of three viruses: HIV (6 percent), hepatitis B (5 percent), or hepatitis C (18 percent). Eighty-three percent of the intravenous drug users, 21 percent of the people who had transfusions, and 21 percent of the homosexual male patients had hepatitis C. Of all the patients who were bleeding and who had invasive procedures performed, 30 percent had at least one virus.

This study shows the potential exposure of medical personnel to hepatitis C infection. HIV testing alone failed to identify 87 percent of those who had hepatitis B and 80 percent of patients with hepatitis C.

> *When I started my career as a medical technician, I got a needle stick. They gave me gamma globulin, but the supply was tainted until 1990. Then two years ago, they detected hepatitis C. I was really sick with infected fluid in my legs, and I was hemorrhaging. They gave me 25 units of blood.*
>
> *Out of five people in our lab, three ended up with hepatitis C, but mine is the only one that became active. My doctor calls it "a thief in the night."*

Erica

Fortunately, the risk of acquiring hepatitis C after a needle stick is relatively low. In two studies with a total of 201 cases of needle-stick accidents involving hepatitis C patients, transmission occurred in only 5 percent.

The best measure of virus in the blood is HCV-RNA (see Chapter 2, PCR assays). None of the RNA-negative patients transmitted HCV to the staff, but seven cases (10 percent) of hepatitis C developed in medical personnel who got the needle stick from an RNA-positive patient. These limited results suggest that health care workers receiving needle sticks from RNA-positive patients are at greatest risk.

More and more state laws and recent Department of Labor Occupational Safety & Health Administration (OSHA) directives now require the use of safe needle technology. Worldwide, unsafe injection practices cause an estimated 2.3 to 4.7 million hepatitis C infections a year. The World Health Organization and other partners have formed the Safe Injection Global Network (SIGN) to tackle the problem.

How do we treat a person who has a needle-stick accident? No one has conducted a well-studied approach to treatment. Although immune serum globulin is commonly administered, we haven't proven its ability to prevent hepatitis C. In contrast, interferon may be useful in preventing the hepatitis from becoming chronic.

I currently recommend that all individuals sustaining a needle stick from an HCV antibody-positive patient be monitored in the following ways: ALT monthly for six months; HCV-Ab (EIA2) at baseline, six months, and 12 months. People who develop elevated ALT or positive HCV antibody should undergo RNA testing and be considered for treatment.

Tattooing and Body Piercing

Tattooing and body piercing are ancient rites in many cultures. In this country, we're witnessing a recent surge of interest in "body art." The practice of tattooing is particularly common in the military and among gang members and prisoners. It's also becoming an accepted cosmetic practice.

Celebrities have popularized the trend. Comedian Roseanne and ex-husband Tom Arnold had each other's names tattooed on their backsides. Famous athletes have decorated their bodies, including Mike Peluso's tattoo of the Stanley Cup and Steve Everitt's bleeding dagger. Unfortunately, even the most benign-appearing tattooing may have its dark side (see Figure 3A). Viral hepatitis, mainly hepatitis B, is the best-documented infection transmitted by tattoos in the 20th century. Two epidemiologic studies implicate tattooing in the transmission of hepatitis C.

FIGURE 3A: HEPATITIS C PATIENT WITH TATTOO

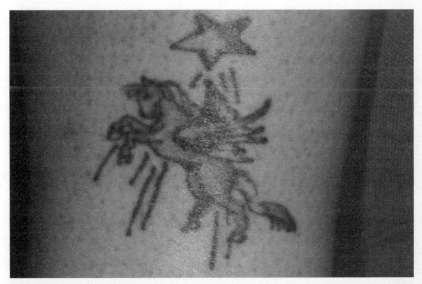

LEGEND 3A: This seemingly innocuous tattoo may have been a source of transmission of hepatitis C to this patient.

Here's a switch. I'm a tattoo artist, and last year I found out I have
hepatitis C. I have antibodies to hepatitis B, too. My joints hurt so much
I can't work. I feel like I'm sliding down the evolutionary scale, because
I can't move my opposable thumbs.

I'm sure I got hepatitis from a needle stick. Fifteen years ago, who
wore gloves?

Peter

Nine percent of males and 1 percent of females in the United States
get tattoos—with peak ages between 14 and 22. And tattoos are common in certain groups at high risk for hepatitis C and other viral infections: intravenous drug abusers, gang members, prostitutes, and
prisoners. In one study 65 percent of prisoners had tattoos.

This flag on my arm—I was young and in the Navy. What did I
know? Now I'm told that there are certified tattoo artists, and if you go
to someone reputable, everything is sterilized.

Well, too late for me. It wasn't like that in Hong Kong.

Jerry

Tattooing involves shaving the skin, placing ink on it, then pushing
the ink through the skin with a needle gun. A small amount of bleeding
is common. The problem is that sterilization techniques vary, and home-
tattooing kits may contain inadequate methods for sterilization. Other
problems encountered with tattoo techniques are lack of disposable needles and repeated insertion of tattoo needles into potentially contaminated ink, which is then re-used on other clients.

Body piercing of the earlobes, nose, lips, and other areas also breaks
the skin. Therefore, the principles and risk of transmission of hepatitis C
are the same as in tattooing.

Resource: The Alliance for Professional Tattooists (APT) has developed a set of infection control guidelines in association with the FDA for
its members. For a copy of "Basic Guidelines for Getting a Tattoo," email
info@safetattoos.com or access its website: www.safetattoos.com/faq.
htm.

Sharing Sharp Instruments

Family and friends who live with hepatitis C patients don't appear to have an increased risk of getting the virus. Nonetheless, you should take care to prevent your blood, which contains hepatitis C, from inoculating another person accidentally.

> *Yesterday I found my oldest son, a teenager, standing in front of the bathroom mirror and trying to shave for the first time. I got so scared. My husband has hepatitis C.*
>
> *Why didn't we see how fast our son was growing? Why didn't we warn him not to borrow his dad's razor?*
>
> *Jan*

Talk to family members and explain why it's important to avoid sharing razor blades, nail clippers, scissors, and toothbrushes. These measures are just good hygiene; it's also sensible to bandage any cuts or abrasions and to safely dispose of menstrual pads and tampons.

In my clinical experience I have seen only one case where transmission of viral hepatitis (hepatitis B, in this instance) from brother to sister occurred because they commonly shared a shaving razor blade.

Birth and Delivery

If you have hepatitis C and you're pregnant or planning a family, of course you're concerned about giving birth to a healthy baby. The period of risk occurs at delivery when the mother's and baby's blood may become intermixed. Mothers with hepatitis C who are otherwise healthy rarely transmit the virus to their newborns. The chance of transmitting hepatitis C from mother to baby at the time of delivery is approximately 6 percent. In contrast, mothers with HIV who are also infected with hepatitis C may transmit hepatitis C to their babies 15 percent or more of the time.

Mothers with hepatitis C often ask whether they can transmit the virus to their baby through breastfeeding. Current studies do not allow us to draw a definite conclusion. However, existing information suggests that hepatitis C is rarely—if ever—transmitted to an infant through breast milk. Even though hepatitis C may be detected in breast milk, it's likely that the baby's digestive juices and enzymes would destroy the virus (see Chapter 13).

Sexual Transmission

This is one of the most sensitive and troubling topics for patients. The risk of getting hepatitis C through sexual contact is minimal, but some spouses are wary. Trust dissolves, the gap widens, and the couple can end up in divorce court.

It's just as hard for singles. How do you start an intimate relationship without being honest about hepatitis C? And how will the other person react?

> *I'm single, and I'm not the smoothest, slickest character around. It's always been hard for me to meet women. Now I have to tell them I have hepatitis C. When should I tell them? Will they want to have anything to do with me?*
>
> *Russ*

> *I'm feeling low, depressed. I was dating this guy, and the relationship was going well. It felt right. Then he broke up with me two days ago. I'm trying not to be paranoid—I mean it could have happened anyway—but he broke up with me a week after I told him I had hepatitis C.*
>
> *Nancy*

Perhaps some solid information will help you come to grips with this issue. Compared to hepatitis B, hepatitis C circulates in your blood at relatively low levels. It is either not detected or found in low concentrations in body fluids, such as saliva, urine, feces, semen, or vaginal secretions.

The vast majority of sexual partners of patients with hepatitis C tests negative for hepatitis C. When a sexual partner does test positive, in most cases this partner has had other risk factors for acquiring hepatitis C, such as intravenous drug use or exposure to blood or blood products. In a study of selected couples without other risk factors, no case of sexual transmission of hepatitis C occurred—even after a calculated 713 person-years of exposure. In contrast, epidemiological studies suggest a higher risk. In my opinion, heterosexual transmission of hepatitis C is rare in a stable, single-partner relationship.

Sally's diagnosis shocked us. We were completely naive. She worried about giving me hepatitis C until we learned more and got a pretty good handle on it.

We've been cautious, but it's not like I'm terrified to go near her. We've been together six years, and I saw no reason to treat her differently or to change our behavior, because I was already exposed.

Sally felt dirty. I did everything I could to diffuse that. It didn't affect the way I felt about her. I kissed her the day before the diagnosis, so why not kiss her the day after?

Ken

My husband got completely paranoid. When I first found out I had hepatitis C, I wanted him to say, "We'll get through this together," but he didn't. He was really nice for a week, then he started getting hostile. He couldn't handle it. I think a big part of it was that we were getting conflicting information about whether or not you can transmit the virus sexually.

We were having troubles before—and I guess the added strain was too much. During my fifth month of interferon, he left me and our three-year-old daughter.

Danielle

Sexual transmission of hepatitis C may be more frequent in homosexual males or highly promiscuous heterosexuals. Some sexual practices are more traumatic to body tissues. For example, anal intercourse may disrupt the lining of the rectum and allow blood, containing hepatitis C, to enter the blood of a sexual partner.

Organ Transplantation

Can a person get hepatitis C from a transplanted organ? Yes, if the donor has hepatitis C, the virus will infect the recipient of the donor organ. Two studies address this issue.

In one study, 28 percent of patients who received organs from donors with hepatitis C developed clinical evidence of liver disease during a follow-up period ranging from three months to six-and-a-half years. In a second study, all the recipients who did not have hepatitis C before the transplant, and who received an organ from a hepatitis C donor, developed hepatitis C after the transplant.

In the University of Colorado liver transplant program, we restrict the use of organs from hepatitis C patients to two situations: recipients already infected with hepatitis C or recipients in desperate medical condition who are awaiting a donor organ at the highest urgency status (hospitalized on life support and not likely to survive seven days without a transplant).

Can you, as a hepatitis C patient, donate an organ for transplanting? Yes. Even though you have hepatitis C, you may still be able to donate your organs for transplant. The organs most commonly used are the kidney and liver, but only if the liver shows no active disease or scarring.

How Can I Avoid Infecting Others?

My patients often inquire about protecting friends and family from the virus. Here are some common questions people ask:

Is it okay to kiss and hug my kids? Yes, you can kiss and hug your children, and they can kiss and hug you back. There is no data to suggest that you could infect your children by these actions.

Should I have members of my family tested for hepatitis C? The risk of transmission from you to other family members, including your spouse, is very low through casual contact and heterosexual activity and, in general, testing is not necessary. If your spouse or child has elevated liver enzyme tests, then they should be tested for hepatitis C. Children of infected mothers should be tested. If family members had any blood-to-blood contact, they should be tested.

Can I cook for my family? What if I cut myself while I'm preparing food? Certainly you can cook for your family. Even if you cut yourself and get blood in the food, it's unlikely that anyone eating the food will get hepatitis C. The enzymes in the digestive tract will destroy or inactivate the virus.

What if my child or friend eats food off my plate or uses my fork? You don't transmit hepatitis C by sharing drinks or food. Hepatitis C is transmitted by contaminated blood entering your bloodstream—not your stomach.

In some Asian cultures, caregivers pre-chew food for babies. It is hypothetically possible to transmit hepatitis C through saliva if the chewer and baby have mouth sores or bloody gums. Sharing of toothbrushes and anything else that might come in contact with blood or body fluids can also expose people to the same hypothetical risks. Even though these are not common or likely infection routes, it makes good common sense to avoid such behaviors for hygienic reasons.

My teenager borrowed my manicure scissors. Is that a problem? I recommend that you avoid sharing sharp instruments. There is a possibility that if your teenager cut herself on your scissors, she could inoculate herself with blood you might have left on the scissors. It's best to avoid sharing all sharp instruments, such as nail clippers, razor blades, toothbrushes, etc.

We've been married for 15 years. Is it safe to have sex? The existing information indicates that sexual transmission between individuals in a stable, single partner, monogamous relationship rarely—if ever—occurs. In addition, people involved in a stable relationship do not need to alter their sexual practices.

I'm single. What should I tell my dates? If you're heterosexual and involved with one partner, my sense is the sexual transmission is so low that it may not be an issue. On the other hand, you have a trust issue that you have to resolve; that may require disclosing your hepatitis C infection. Place the disclosure in the context of knowing that your hepatitis C infection need not fracture or destroy an otherwise promising relationship. Infected males may provide additional protection for their female sexual partners by using latex condoms.

What about French kissing? Oral sex? The details of these types of sexual activity have not been scientifically investigated. If blood barriers (lining of the mouth, lining of the genitalia) are breached, then blood-to-blood transmission may occur.

Should I always use condoms? Latex condoms and safe sex practices are especially suggested for individuals who have multiple sex partners.

Can I have a baby? Nurse my baby? Yes. Mothers who ask these questions are worried about transmitting hepatitis C to their infants.

First, the risk of transmission appears to be limited to the time of delivery, when the blood of the mother and infant may become intermixed. Approximately 6 percent of babies born of mothers with hepatitis C develop the infection.

As stated above, swallowing mother's milk is not likely to be harmful to the infant. (For more information, see Chapter 13.) Always discuss these decisions with your doctor.

How do I clean up a blood spill? If you have gloves available, use them. If not, take precautions to prevent contact of the blood with your skin or any cuts, abrasions, sores, or wounds on your skin. Take a rag or paper cloth and wipe the spill. If household bleach is available, use diluted bleach at the site of the spill. Dispose of the rag or paper in a plastic bag, and throw it in the garbage. Wash your hands afterwards. The term "Universal Precautions" when dealing with potentially infectious matter means to wear gloves, avoid exposure to infection, and wash your hands.

Is it necessary to tell people like my dentist that I have hepatitis C? In my opinion, patients should inform dentists and other health care professionals who need to perform invasive procedures or operations.

Can I be an organ donor? Yes. Some organs from hepatitis C patients are used, particularly for recipients who are critically ill or who already have hepatitis C.

We learn geology the morning after the earthquake.

Emerson

Reference

1. Alter, Harvey J., C. Conry-Cantilena, J. Melpolder, D. Tan, M. Van Raden, D. Herion, D. Lau, J.H. Hoofnagle, "Hepatitis C in Asymptomatic Blood Donors," *Hepatology* 1997;26(Suppl 1):295-335.

4

LEARNING ABOUT YOUR LIVER: YOUR BODY'S CHEMICAL FACTORY

Liver Facts and Liver Disease Symptoms

from Oda al Higado (Ode to the Liver)[1]
by Pablo Neruda

> *. . . navigating*
> *the hidden mysteries,*
> *the alchemist's chamber*
> *of life's microscopic,*
> *echoic, inner oceans . . .*

Translated by Herberto Morales and Will Hochman

IMAGINE A MACHINE that converts food into energy; stores nutrients, fats, and vitamins; makes proteins for blood plasma; and detoxifies poisons. Your liver does all this and more—much more.

But no machine, no matter how powerful, is as versatile as your liver. Even if 75 percent of the liver's mass is taken away, it still functions. And it's the only internal organ that regenerates itself.

This chapter will discuss what the liver looks like, how it functions, and what happens to the liver when it's infected with hepatitis C— including ten warning signals your body sends you when liver function is compromised:

• Liver Facts from Mesopotamian to Modern Times
• A Look at Your Liver
   Appearance
   Under the Microscope
• How Your Liver Works
   Blood
   Bile
   Lymph
   Immune System
   Chemical Factory
   Bilirubin
   ALT, AST, GGT, Alkaline Phosphatase
   Albumin
   Clotting Factors
   Hormones
• Phases of Hepatitis C
   Phase I: Infection
   Phase II: Inflammation
   Phase III: Fibrosis
   Phase IV: Cirrhosis
• Ten Danger Signs of Liver Disease
   Early Warning Signs: #1–#2
   Early Symptoms
   Changes in Liver Functions
   Later Warning Signs of Cirrhosis: #3–#10
   Compensated Cirrhosis
   Decompensated Cirrhosis
   Changes in the Appearance of the Skin: Jaundice, Spider Nevi
      (Telangiectasia), Palmar Erythema
   Fluid Buildup: Ascites

    Bleeding: Variceal Hemorrhage
    Mental Confusion: Encephalopathy
    Weight Loss
    Thinning of Bones (Osteoporosis) and Fractures:
        Metabolic Bone Disease
    Blood Clotting Problems: Coagulopathy
    Itching: Pruritus
• Beyond the Liver: Conditions Associated with Hepatitis C
    Kidney Damage
    Cryoglobulinemia
    Thyroid Disease
    Skin Conditions
    Autoimmune Conditions

Liver Facts from Mesopotamian to Modern Times

- Mesopotamians didn't know anatomy, but they could see that the liver seemed to be the collecting point for blood, the source of life. Archeologists have found 5,000-year-old Mesopotamian clay models of livers with markings that may have helped priests perform religious rites.
- In ancient cultures, animals were sacrificed before battle and their entrails were examined; a healthy blood-red liver was a good omen. Pale livers foretold defeat—an expression that has entered the English language with the term "lily-livered," meaning cowardly.
- In Greek mythology, Prometheus stole fire from the gods and gave it to mankind. Zeus punished him by chaining him to a rock in the mountains. Each day an eagle gnawed at his body, feasting on his liver. Because the liver has such great regenerating capacity, it grew back each night, subjecting Prometheus to an endless ordeal.
- In 1987, a granite sculpture of the liver was unveiled in Ferrol, Spain. The city's coroner, who doubled as the mayor, said that over the years he saw "hundreds of these organs tortured by cocktails, wine, tranquilizers, and other medications . . . but every day, the poor little liver is at work neutralizing and purifying everything we take in."[2] As the monument was dedicated, a local poet recited "Oda Al Higado" (Ode to the Liver) by the late Nobel prize-winner, Pablo Neruda.

A Look at Your Liver

Appearance. As a hepatologist, a doctor who studies livers, I sometimes forget that my patients usually don't have a clear idea of what this organ looks like. Here's Hedy:

> *As a kid, I hated the sight of blood, never looked at body charts in encyclopedias, and avoided first aid classes. In short, I didn't know where my liver was. Right side or left? High in my chest or low in my gut?*
>
> *I worried about every ache and pain, sure my condition was getting worse by the minute. So I went to the library and took out some children's books with terrific diagrams and simple explanations.*
>
> *Finally, I believed my doctor. What I was feeling was heartburn, pure and simple. Learning more about my liver helped me reduce stress and, incidentally, the heartburn.*

Learning more about your liver can give you a greater feeling of control and reduce stress, so let's examine this organ—the largest one in your body. The liver weighs about three pounds in an adult male and sits in the upper right of the abdomen, protected by the rib cage (see Figure 4A).

If you've ever gone to the supermarket or butcher, you've seen animal livers. They give you a pretty good idea of what the human liver looks and feels like. Reddish-brown in color, it's shaped like a flattened football with two lobes. The larger lobe lies closest to your right side. The liver is surrounded by vital organs: diaphragm and lungs above, kidney behind, intestine and colon below.

Major blood vessels serve as conduits to deliver blood to and from the liver. Your blood system transports food, oxygen, and waste. Because your liver is a central depot for so many body functions, it has the largest and most complex blood supply of any organ in the body. In fact, about 1.5 quarts of blood flow through the liver every minute.

Like other parts of your body, the liver has an artery to supply it with oxygenated blood (the hepatic artery via the abdominal aorta) and hepatic veins to take blood back to the heart. The hepatic veins join the inferior vena cava, the major vein just below the diaphragm.

In addition to the hepatic artery, the liver has a second source of blood, the portal vein. This vein is responsible for at least two-thirds of

FIGURE 4A. ANATOMIC LOCATION OF THE LIVER IN HUMANS

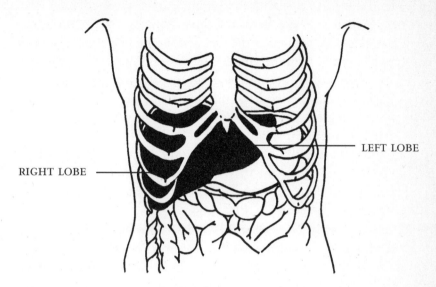

RIGHT LOBE

LEFT LOBE

LEGEND 4A: The liver is located in the right upper quadrant of the abdomen and is protected from external trauma by the rib cage.

liver blood flow and delivers nutrients and toxins absorbed by the intestine to the liver for processing.

Have you ever wondered why livers are a dull red color? It's because the portal vein transports nutrients to the liver in dark, deoxygenated blood.

Speaking of colors, your liver produces up to a quart a day of yellow-green bile, a liquid that looks like motor oil and breaks down fat in foods. Bile flows from the liver into the bile duct, which resembles the branches of a tree. The smallest branches are embedded in the liver while the common bile duct is the tree "trunk."

The common bile duct connects with the gallbladder (which stores bile and is attached to the underside of your liver) through the cystic duct. Then the bile duct continues through the pancreas, where it's joined by the pancreatic duct, and on to the intestine.

Under the Microscope. Tiny units, called lobules, are the building blocks of your liver tissue. Each lobule is a spheroid structure and measures about 0.2 inches across. Under the microscope, you see flat sheets of cube-shaped liver cells (hepatocytes) fanning out from a tiny central vein. Blood flows in the spaces (sinusoids) between the sheets.

Small branches of the hepatic artery (bringing oxygen from the heart) and the portal vein enter the lobule from the side and first deliver blood to the periphery of the lobule (portal area). Blood travels through the lobule toward its center, bathing the hepatocytes with nutrients, chemicals and toxins carried from the intestine. Liver cells have special ways of extracting compounds from blood and metabolizing them—a topic I'll talk about in the next section.

The center of the lobule contains a very fine terminal branch of the hepatic vein. This vein then connects with other branches and "processed" blood flows through the hepatic veins to the inferior vena cava, returning to the heart.

In addition, each liver cell makes and secretes bile to its own tiny attached branch of the biliary system. The liver contains a whole network of these fine tubes that pipe bile to the bile duct and gallbladder.

How Your Liver Works

Knowing how the liver works will help you understand why things go wrong when a virus attacks it. Your liver affects your blood, bile, lymph, immune system, and chemical functions.

Blood. The liver greatly influences the makeup of blood in your body. Blood is composed of plasma (a liquid), red cells, white cells, and platelets. When the liver is diseased, all of these blood components may be affected.

Do you know how your body tissues get oxygen? Red blood cells deliver it. Do you know why wounds clot? Platelets plug bleeding capillaries and vessels. When you have an infection, white blood cells rush to the site as your first line of defense.

The liver receives blood from two sources: two-thirds from the portal vein (which comes from the intestine loaded with nutrients for the liver to process) and one-third from the hepatic artery. The hepatic artery, like all arteries, carries blood loaded with oxygen. About 15 percent of the blood pumped by the heart each minute runs through the liver.

As the liver becomes progressively injured, scar tissue builds up, making it difficult for blood from the portal vein and hepatic artery to flow through the liver. The blood tends to back up into other abdominal vessels and the spleen. As blood backs up in the spleen, cells become trapped and are destroyed—resulting in a decrease in platelets, red cells, and white cells.

Bile. Did you know that cholesterol is an ingredient in bile? Your liver makes bile from water, electrolytes (sodium, potassium, chloride, and others), proteins, organic salts (bilirubin), and lipids (cholesterol, among others). The liver turns compounds that don't dissolve in water into water-soluble substances that are secreted into bile. Toxins (poisons) absorbed from the intestine also circulate in blood to the liver, which extracts, inactivates, and secretes them into bile.

Back to cholesterol. A normal part of our diets, it's made by several cells in our bodies. When too much cholesterol accumulates, cells may alter their functions and even die. If too much cholesterol builds up in blood vessels, you may get hardening of the arteries (atherosclerosis). If it builds up in bile, you may develop gallstones.

Prevention of these complications depends on eliminating excess cholesterol. Your liver is the only organ that breaks down cholesterol into bile acid, secretes it in bile, and removes it from your body for good.

What else does bile do? Simply put, bile helps you absorb fat and vitamins that are dissolved in fat (A, D, E, and K). When disease interrupts this cycle, your body has trouble digesting and absorbing fats and fat-soluble vitamins and getting rid of pigments and toxins. Processing of medications may also be impaired if your liver is severely damaged, and your doctor may need to adjust the doses of your medications.

Lymph. Your liver produces about a quart of lymph a day. Filtered from plasma, it's a protein-rich fluid composed mostly of water and electrolytes. Lymph travels through channels next to the portal vein and joins other major lymph channels in the abdomen. Eventually, the lymph is dumped into the bloodstream.

Any kind of disruption, whether it's disease or congestion of the lymph channels, may mean that large amounts of lymph spill into the abdomen. Although this rarely happens, it may be one reason for swelling of the abdomen due to fluid (ascites).

Immune System. Here's a mouthful: lymphocytes, plasma cells, macrophages, fibroblasts, dendritic cells, and polymorphonuclear leucocytes. All types of immune cells, including these, are found in the liver. In fact, the liver is one of the major lymphoid organs of the immune system.

The immune cells in the liver protect against infections or toxins, but may also, in certain diseases, cause liver injury. In hepatitis C, liver damage is caused not only by the direct effects of the virus but also by the immune response to the virus.

Chemical Factory. Your liver acts as a chemical powerhouse—building the substances you need for life and neutralizing or safely dumping harmful material. In fact, your liver performs more than 500 complex chemical functions!

I hope you're beginning to see that your liver works overtime to help and protect you. Take your digestive system, for instance. The liver stores nutrients, then sends them out to the parts of your body that need them.

When you eat carbohydrates (potatoes, pasta, and other starches), your body breaks them down into glucose. You need glucose for energy, but because of your liver, you don't have to eat carbohydrates all day long. Instead, the liver stores glucose as glycogen. When you need a burst of energy, your liver turns glycogen back into glucose and sends it through the bloodstream to your body.

Some of the fats you eat build new cells. The liver sends extra fat into the blood and, eventually, your body stores it as fat cells (adipose tissue). If you run out of carbohydrates, the fat stored in your liver becomes a major source of body fuel.

Protein you eat is broken down in your gut into amino acids, which are absorbed and distributed via the bloodstream to your liver and body. Cells use the amino acids to make new proteins or burn the amino acids for fuel. Proteins made by the liver regulate your clotting system, transport fat and nutrients throughout your body, control hormone levels, and maintain your blood volume.

Bilirubin. Bilirubin is the yellow pigment responsible for jaundice. When red blood cells in your body break down, they release hemoglobin—a molecule that carries oxygen to your tissues.

Enzymes are proteins that make specific chemical reactions take place. One of these enzymes, called heme oxygenase, occurs in bone marrow and liver cells. It converts heme, the major component of hemoglobin, into bilirubin. The liver then removes the bilirubin from your blood and turns it into a water-soluble form that is excreted into bile.

Normally, the amount of bilirubin produced approximates the rate of red blood cell breakdown. Bilirubin levels rise when something goes wrong, such as the breakdown of too many red blood cells, the development of liver disease (such as hepatitis), a defect in liver metabolism, or a blockage of the bile system. Bilirubin accumulates in tissues, causing your skin and the white part of your eyes (sclerae) to turn yellow.

ALT (SGPT), AST (SGOT), GGT, Alkaline Phosphatase. Your liver creates all of these enzymes. When liver cells are injured, the enzymes escape and enter the bloodstream. If small numbers of cells are affected, there may be little or no increase in plasma levels of enzymes. When large numbers of liver cells are injured or die, the levels of these enzymes in plasma increase markedly.

Enzyme tests roughly reflect the level of ongoing injury, but they don't indicate how your liver is actually functioning. To do that, you need to look at the tests that measure your liver's ability to build and synthesize (albumin, clotting factors) or to excrete (bilirubin).

Albumin. The liver makes this protein. It is vital for maintaining body fluid balance, especially the volume of plasma in your blood.

Although albumin levels in plasma may be affected by other disorders, in liver disease the level of serum albumin is a good marker of your liver's ability to produce proteins. A sustained decrease below the normal range is one of the first signs of advancing liver disease.

Clotting Factors. The liver also makes many proteins that help the blood to clot. In contrast to albumin, which stays a long time in plasma, clotting factors have a relatively short survival period. Therefore, the liver must constantly work to produce enough coagulation factors to maintain normal clotting.

When the liver is injured and can't make clotting factors, plasma levels drop within one or two days. Soon patients notice that they're bruising or bleeding easily even after minor bumps and injuries. If liver failure occurs, patients may hemorrhage and often require plasma and blood transfusions.

Hormones. The thyroid is one of the main hormone-producing glands. Patients with chronic hepatitis C have a high occurrence of underlying thyroid disease. Interferon therapy may cause the thyroid condition to flare. Therefore, doctors commonly run tests for thyroid function before and after interferon treatment.

In late stages of liver disease (cirrhotic phase), patients may experience other hormonal imbalances, including altered ovulation or gonadal function and impairment of the pituitary gland (the main hormone control center). For example, men with cirrhosis often develop distressing enlargement of their breasts due to hormonal imbalance. In addition, pituitary hormones regulate functions such as sleep-wake cycles, appetite, and body temperature.

> *My wife kept nagging me to tell the doctor how sore the nipple was on my right breast. "But what if it's cancer?" she said. At my next office visit, I worked up the nerve to ask.*
> *"Hormones change in end-stage liver disease," my doctor said.*
> *"Are you telling me what I think you are?"*
> *"Yes," he said. "You're growing a breast."*
> *I couldn't believe it. Cowboys don't grow breasts!*
>
> *Larry*

FIGURE 4B. CONSEQUENCES OF HCV INFECTION

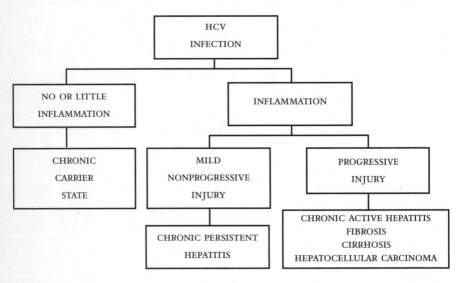

LEGEND 4B: Potential consequences of hepatitis C infection are shown. Some patients develop no or very little inflammation and co-exist with hepatitis C in a chronic carrier state. Others experience variable degrees of inflammation and liver damage. In the most severe cases, scarring becomes severe, resulting in cirrhosis or liver cancer (hepatocellular carcinoma—hepatoma).

Phases of Hepatitis C

Figure 4B diagrams the consequences of hepatitis C infection. We divide hepatitis C infection and disease into four overlapping phases:

I. Infection
II. Inflammation
III. Fibrosis
IV. Cirrhosis

Phase I: Infection. When the hepatitis C virus gets into the bloodstream, it attaches to liver cells, enters them, and starts to reproduce. The new virus, made within the infected liver cell, exits into the bloodstream where it attaches to and infects another liver cell. This process allows the infection to spread through the liver.

Patients often ask me, "Why do I have hepatitis C if I have antibodies against hepatitis C?" Although your body produces an immune response to the virus (antibodies form and immune cells called lymphocytes are recruited into the liver), it usually doesn't get rid of the infection. We now know that approximately 85 percent of patients become chronically infected. In other infections antibodies effectively fight the infection, but in hepatitis C the antibodies are ineffective and do not clear the infection. In fact, antibodies (when present) usually indicate active disease and ongoing infection.

Phase II: Inflammation. In this phase, liver inflammation (hepatitis) develops. Under the microscope, most liver cells appear relatively normal and uninjured. But in some areas there is liver cell injury and death. Inflammation in the liver is characterized by the presence of specific immune cells called lymphocytes. Lymphocytes are recruited to the liver to attempt to eliminate hepatitis C. However, they also release chemicals that damage liver cells and contribute to the liver injury.

In the majority of cases, the initial, acute phase of hepatitis C is mild in terms of symptoms. Most people don't realize they've had a first attack, and there are only a few cases of sudden, severe (fulminant) liver failure due to the virus. Most patients have no symptoms and only a fraction develop jaundice.

We now know that most patients with hepatitis C will develop chronic hepatitis. The chronic form, too, is usually mild and asymptomatic, although many patients complain of fatigue, poor stamina, and inability to concentrate.

Phase III: Fibrosis. Despite the mild nature of the inflammation and liver injury, the disease commonly progresses to fibrosis—the formation of scar tissue in the liver. If your liver biopsy shows significant fibrosis, it usually means you've had hepatitis C for more than 10 years.

Phase IV: Cirrhosis. When fibrosis increases, the fourth stage appears. With cirrhosis, the fibrosis is so severe that it affects how the liver functions and grossly distorts the architecture and blood flow of the liver.

Ten Danger Signs of Liver Disease

Warning symptoms fall into two categories: early and late. The liver sends few early warning signs. It's a large organ with great reserve; most people can lose three-quarters of their liver without any change in function or development of symptoms.

In early hepatitis C, even though the liver is damaged, no symptoms appear. Symptoms early in the course of hepatitis C, such as muscle aches and headaches, are due to the virus itself and not to liver failure. Later in the course of hepatitis C, liver function diminishes and warning signs of advanced liver disease appear.

Early Warning Signs: #1–#2

#1: Early Symptoms. Here's Hedy:

> At our hepatitis C support group, we compared notes. No one had serious symptoms like itching or mental confusion, even though one of us had cirrhosis. Almost everyone, however, complained of fatigue.
>
> It also turned out that four of us often experienced a kind of tender, achy feeling on our right sides. Doctors had dismissed the symptom by saying the liver didn't feel pain—not to worry. But of course, we did.
>
> So at my next medical appointment, I brought up the mystery symptom and got an answer. The liver doesn't feel pain, but the membrane around the liver and the liver itself may react to the inflammation from hepatitis.
>
> I reported back to the group, and we all relaxed. Nothing had changed, but the simple explanation helped. It kept us from imagining that we were sliding into liver failure.

Many people with hepatitis C, especially in the early phases, tell me they have no symptoms. I find, however, that if I question them closely, they complain of fatigue, feel less energetic, and are unable to work at their usual high level. Typically, appetite and weight are unaffected, but occasionally some patients report less enthusiasm for eating and so have difficulty maintaining their weight.

No one knows why these common symptoms occur. Some researchers think they're due to the viral infection itself, while others feel that the ongoing liver injury releases substances into the blood that produce these effects.

In my experience, these symptoms rarely, if at all, correspond to the severity of the disease. Some of my patients suffer extreme fatigue but have little injury to their livers, while others with aggressive hepatitis and cirrhosis may have no symptoms at all.

#2: Changes in Liver Functions. If you have hepatitis C, you need close medical supervision. Current recommendations call for an annual physical exam and liver blood tests every six months. Changes in blood tests usually pick up the first sign of deteriorating liver function.

> *Twenty-four years ago I had a really bad car accident, lost part of my liver, and had last rites. I received lots of blood transfusions. Afterwards, it was really weird. I got so tired I could barely mow my lawn.*
>
> *Finally, I was diagnosed with hepatitis C. I was back in school, and right after graduation my blood tests changed. My bilirubin was up, so I was a little jaundiced. My platelet count was really low—one-third what it was supposed to be. Platelets coagulate your blood, so if I barely bumped something, my skin would tear, and I'd bleed. My nose was bleeding all the time.*
>
> *Pete*

At later stages of disease, albumin may decrease, bilirubin may rise, and prothrombin (a protein involved in blood clotting) time may increase. These changes occur because the liver is becoming less able to make its usual quota of substances the body needs. Another change that occurs is enlargement of the spleen. Platelets, white blood cells, and even red blood cells may drop because the enlarged spleen traps and destroys these cells. In my experience, a progressive buildup of fluid in the ankles and a low level of sodium in the blood are also common. These danger signs correlate with the cirrhotic stage. They indicate that the liver is less able to keep up with the amount of injury and often precede more serious symptoms of liver failure.

Later Warning Signs of Cirrhosis: #3–#10

What does cirrhosis mean? Cirrhosis simply means the hardening of the liver due to a buildup of scar tissue and formation of nodules.

Compensated Cirrhosis. Patients who have early-stage cirrhosis, also known as compensated cirrhosis, may not have any symptoms or laboratory test abnormalities.

Decompensated Cirrhosis. Late-stage cirrhosis, or decompensated cirrhosis, is characterized by abnormalities in blood tests, complications (some of which are life threatening), and limited survival. Patients with any or all of the following signs may be potential candidates for a liver transplant.

#3: Changes in the Appearance of the Skin: Jaundice, Spider Nevi (Telangiectasia), Palmar Erythema.

Jaundice. Jaundice is the yellowing of the skin and whites of the eyes. It is due to an accumulation of the pigment bilirubin in the skin and other tissues of the body, such as the whites of the eyes. Jaundice commonly occurs in patients with hepatitis C when the liver disease is advanced and the hepatitis flares. In some cases, jaundice may disappear when the flare resolves.

> *I was like the walking dead. My skin was a poor color—gray. Other days, I was yellow, jaundiced. I didn't think I was going to make it, but I did. The transplant worked, and I'm grateful.*
>
> *Blaire*

Spider Nevi (Telangiectasia). Spider nevi are red spots, usually on the upper body and face. If you look at the spots closely, you will see a central red area with fine red lines emanating outward. These "spiders" are actually a collection of very small blood vessels caused by hormonal imbalance due to cirrhosis. The spiders disappear after transplantation.

Palmar Erythema. Palmar erythema is a reddening of the fleshy part of the palms of the hands. The condition occurs when blood vessels dilate because of hormonal imbalance due to cirrhosis. Palmar erythema and spider nevi often occur simultaneously.

#4: Fluid Buildup: Ascites. Ascites means that fluid builds up in the abdomen, so that the belly swells. Liver disease is the most common cause of ascites.

> *I didn't realize I was holding water. I thought, "What have I eaten that's made my stomach so bloated?" At one point the doctor figured I was carrying 30 to 35 pounds of water in my stomach.*
>
> *The swelling came and went, but in the last year it's been an acute problem. My fingers, knees, even my calves are swollen. My skin is so tight that my feet look like little porky pigs. The doctor gives me diuretics to make me go to the bathroom. It makes for a busy day!*
>
> *Jerry*

> *If I eat too much, the ascites gets worse. A huge meal does me in. Afterwards, I feel like I'm going to explode! The best thing is to eat in small amounts, a little bit at a time.*
>
> *Josie*

Physicians must remove and analyze the fluid to exclude other causes. To remove fluid the physician performs a paracentesis, which involves placing a needle through the abdominal wall and drawing out the fluid for a culture, cell count, biochemical tests, and a microscopic examination. If the ascites is due to liver disease, the fluid will be clear, yellow, uninfected, and have a low cell count.

More than one problem, however, may be involved. Sometimes patients have a bacterial infection in the ascites (spontaneous bacterial peritonitis). In these cases, there are other signs of infection: fever, high white blood count, abdominal pain. It's important to recognize this condition right away and treat it early with antibiotics. We now have many treatments for ascites, including diuretics (drugs that increase the amount of urine excreted), paracentesis (drawing off fluid), or shunts (tubes that redirect the liquid), such as peritoneovenous shunts and transjugular intrahepatic portal-systemic shunts.

Muscle cramps are a common problem in patients with advanced liver disease. In particular, patients with ascites who are treated with diuretics commonly complain of severe cramping. This type of cramping may respond to reducing diuretics or administering magnesium, calcium, or possibly zinc.

Ascites is a serious warning sign of very advanced liver disease, and most patients with ascites will require a liver transplant for prolonged survival.

#5: Bleeding: Variceal Hemorrhage. The most dramatic and urgent complication of advanced liver disease is variceal hemorrhage. "Variceal" refers to varices, which are abnormally distended or swollen veins usually located in the esophagus, and "hemorrhage," of course, means bleeding.

Patients vomit large quantities of red blood, show signs of altered mental status, and have very low blood pressure. By the time they get to the emergency room, they may be in shock.

> *I didn't know I had hepatitis C until I went into the hospital with an esophageal bleed. It was in 1991. We were having a family picnic, and I had drunk lots of cherry Kool-Aid®. I tried to convince myself the red stuff coming out of my mouth was the punch, but then I bled again. The doctors tubed me through my nose and stopped the bleeding.*
>
> *Chris*

It's urgent to get to an emergency medical facility when there's any sign of bleeding from the upper gastrointestinal tract. Variceal bleeding may be vomiting red blood, the passage of loose, dark, tarry feces, or the passage of a large amount of red blood through the rectum.

Doctors first must find the source of the bleeding before they can treat the problem. They insert a slender tube (endoscope) down the patient's throat to diagnose the cause or source of the bleed. Endoscopists have two treatments available: tying the bleeding veins with bands (ligation) or injecting a chemical into the vein to make it clot (sclerotherapy). Both therapies work well to control the initial bleed. But to eradicate the varices and avoid later hemorrhages, outpatient treatments must be repeated—usually two or three times.

Doctors may also give medications such as somatostatin, vasopressin, nitroglycerin, and plasma products to control the bleeding. Sometimes propranolol or related medicines are given to lower the risk of a rebleed.

Occasionally, varices are also found in the stomach, duodenum, intestine, and colon. It's harder to manage varices in these locations with endoscopic treatment. Doctors often will treat bleeding from these varices with either a surgical shunt (a tube that redirects the blood) or TIPS. Surgical shunts require major abdominal surgery and connect one of the portal veins to veins that bypass the liver (systemic veins).

TIPS is short for transjugular intrahepatic portal-systemic shunt. Radiologists put the TIPS in place, avoiding the need for risky abdominal surgery that might compromise a later liver transplant.

First, the radiologist places a catheter through a vein in the neck, then into the liver via the hepatic veins. A needle goes through this catheter into the liver and punctures a main branch of the portal vein. Once the portal vein and hepatic veins are connected, the radiologist dilates the tract and places an expandable cylindrical wire-mesh shunt across the liver to maintain the connection. When the shunt is in place, it relieves the back pressure on the portal veins, varices collapse, and the risk of further hemorrhage is greatly reduced.

Transplant surgeons welcome TIPS because it doesn't interfere with their surgery. However, occasionally, TIPS migrate into the portal vein and complicate a transplant operation, so most transplant doctors prefer that TIPS be placed by radiologists with a high level of experience with the procedure.

#6: Mental Confusion: Portal-Systemic Encephalopathy. The liver conducts many metabolic functions, including clearing or detoxifying the blood of harmful substances. When the liver fails, these substances may build up to toxic levels and impair the function of other organs, such as the brain.

Just before my liver transplant, my doctors had me take a mental test. They said there were no passing scores, and you couldn't fail—but I did. I flunked it. I know I did.

A year after my transplant, they asked me to take it again. This time I did well. In fact, I did so well, I scored higher than a third of the doctors who took the same test!

Jack

The brain reacts to altered liver functions, so patients with advanced liver disease commonly note changes in their mental abilities. These changes range from slight changes, such as decline in memory or reduced ability to perform complex calculations, to more severe changes, such as confusion, disorientation, blackout spells, or even coma.

It helps to understand four features of encephalopathy: (1) Encephalopathy is usually brought on by some other problem, such as gastrointestinal bleeding, infection, or electrolyte imbalance. (2) It's a completely reversible condition. (3) Effective medical therapy exists [lactulose (a non-absorbable carbohydrate), neomycin (an antibiotic), a protein-restricted diet]. Early therapy may prevent the patient from lapsing into more advanced stages, such as coma. (4) A successful liver transplant completely reverses the condition.

This means that a patient experiencing encephalopathy must get urgent medical attention and evaluation, be treated promptly, and be considered for liver transplantation.

#7: Weight Loss. Because the liver acts as your body's metabolic factory and energy storehouse, advancing liver disease affects your nutrition. That's why your doctor looks for weight loss.

> *I had a lot of muscle because I was a physical therapist. When I look in the mirror now, I can see the wasting. I'm so much thinner in my arms, shoulders, and back. Then again, my stomach's out to here from fluid. So I've got this weird figure.*
>
> *Lila*

Patients need to eat an appropriate amount of calories. And because patients often are on a sodium restriction for ascites and a protein restriction for encephalopathy, that can be hard to do. I usually recommend supplements and a visit to a dietician.

Blood tests detect nutritional deficiencies. People with liver disease, for example, may have fat-soluble vitamin deficiencies (A, D, E, K) that can be at least partially corrected with oral supplements. I prefer retinyl palmitate (vitamin A), Calderol® (vitamin D-25-OH), tocopherol polyethylene glycol solution or TPGS (vitamin E), and Mephyton® (vitamin K). The TPGS formulation of vitamin E is an emulsified liquid that also aids the absorption of A, D, and K. A simple way to think of TPGS is that it's artificial bile. I recommend that all the fat-soluble vitamins be taken with the TPGS to improve absorption.

#8: Thinning of Bones (Osteoporosis) and Fractures: Metabolic Bone Disease. Did you know that as liver disease progresses, bone loss may accelerate? Bone loss is frequently observed in patients with advanced hepatitis C, especially those receiving steroid medication for other conditions.

> *In my whole life I had never broken any bones—pretty unusual. Then in the space of two years, I broke my toe twice. The first time, I fell off my bike; the second, I hit my toe against a floorboard. The final straw came when I fractured my kneecap. Two years later, my knee still aches when the weather changes.*
>
> *Coincidence, growing older, hepatitis C—who knows? But my doctor wants me to take some tests.*
>
> *Sheila*

First, the doctor must exclude other causes of bone loss, such as vitamin D deficiency or hyperparathyroidism. Typically, patients with bone disease and fractures due to end-stage liver disease simply have a condition called osteopenia, which does not respond well to vitamin D, calcium, or fluoride. Recent studies suggest that a new drug, alendronate, may be of some benefit. To complicate matters, post-transplant use of steroids and the relative inactivity after surgery can make the bones more brittle. Most transplant centers now taper steroids sharply and encourage early walking to lower the risk of fractures.

#9: Blood Clotting Problems: Coagulopathy. People with end-stage liver disease have multiple defects in their blood clotting system that put them at risk for bleeding and hemorrhage.

> *Sometimes I just bite into an apple, and I see blood right there—on the fruit. Three times in the last month I woke up with blood in my mouth.*
>
> *Also, I've been getting blood spots—like little red pimples—across my chest and arms. My wife says they look like spider veins. They don't hurt, but if I forget and scratch them, they bleed.*
>
> *Gary*

Coagulation proteins drop to such low levels that even minor trauma to skin, gums, lips or extremities causes marked bruising or prolonged oozing of blood. Major trauma, such as surgery, can result in excessive bleeding. In many cases your doctor may be able to administer clotting factors to reduce your risk of bleeding from these procedures. In addition, the spleen often holds and destroys platelets, reducing the body's other major clotting aid. If severe clotting disturbances develop, it's an ominous sign of advanced liver disease and means immediate consideration for a transplant.

#10: Itching: Pruritus. Although relatively uncommon in patients with hepatitis C, constant itching, day and night, may torment patients with severe jaundice or advanced liver disease. It's caused by a buildup of substances in the skin that are normally cleared by the liver, and it's not associated with hives or rashes (except what people get from scratching). Although generalized, itching may be peculiarly localized to the palms of the hands, soles of the feet, inside the mouth, and the external ear canal.

> *Excuse my language, but I call it "the bitchy itch." My symptoms began as a little itch. I hardly noticed it. I ignored it until it got bigger, and I started scratching. There was one spot the size of a quarter on my left leg. Creams did no good.*
>
> *Over a year-and-a-half it got so bad I swore I'd never scratch—and I've got high will power. But I scarred my legs.*
>
> *Finally, someone in my support group told me to use cornstarch. So now I bathe, dry myself off, and apply the cornstarch. I've done it three times so far, and it helps.*
>
> *Saul*

The pruritus of liver disease does not respond to antihistamines, skin lotions, and creams, but improves with the use of medicines that promote bile flow, such as ursodeoxycholate, or that bind and inactivate substances in the intestine, such as cholestyramine.

Recent studies suggest that pruritus may be related to naturally occurring morphine-like compounds that build up in the patient and may respond to medications that block morphine effects (naloxone, naltrexone).

Some patients have severe, incapacitating pruritus that can't be helped by any of the therapies mentioned. A liver transplant successfully treats the condition.

Beyond the Liver: Conditions Associated with Hepatitis C

The ten danger signs of advanced liver disease and cirrhosis are common to all forms of liver disease, including hepatitis C. In addition, hepatitis C patients may find themselves dealing with other conditions associated with the virus. These conditions are called extra-hepatic (non-liver) manifestations of hepatitis C.

Kidney Damage. A specific type of kidney damage, called glomerulonephritis, can occur when immune complexes of the hepatitis C virus lodge in the kidney and cause inflammation. At first, there may be no symptoms. It's often detected when a routine urinalysis shows protein in the urine. As more protein is lost in urine, the blood albumin may decrease, and patients may notice swelling in the ankles or abdomen. Rarely, it can lead to kidney failure. Glomerulonephritis, complicating hepatitis C, may respond to treatment with interferon.

Cryoglobulinemia. The signs of this condition are skin rash, fever, kidney damage, and ulcerations on the fingers and toes. Cryoglobulinemia is caused by antibodies that the body manufactures against the hepatitis C virus. Management of cryoglobulinemia is complex but may involve interferon, steroids, cyclophosphamide, intravenous immunoglobulins, and plasmapheresis (passing blood through a filter to remove the antibody complexes).

Thyroid Disease. Thyroid disease is very common in the general population (2 to 3 percent) and even more common in hepatitis C patients (5 to 20 percent). Usually, it's an underactive thyroid causing the problem, but in rare cases, the thyroid can be overactive. The signs of an underactive thyroid include cold intolerance, sluggishness, dry skin, coarse hair, a change in voice, mental confusion. Signs of an overactive thyroid include palpitations, sweating, heat intolerance, jitters, tremor, poor concentrating ability, and hypertension.

An underactive thyroid is treated with thyroid hormone replacement, such as levo-thyroxine. Treatment of an overactive thyroid may involve radioactive iodine, beta-blockers, and propylthiouracil.

Skin Conditions. Skin conditions associated with hepatitis C include lichen planus, lichenoid dermatitis, and porphyria cutanea tarda.

The first two are usually best treated with dermatologic lotions/creams and may flare during interferon treatment.

Lichen planus is a reddish-brown raised round spot, typically less than one to two centimeters in diameter. Sometimes it appears scaly and may itch.

Lichenoid dermatitis looks like scaly, reddish flat areas, usually larger than two centimeters in diameter. It's occasionally itchy.

Porphyria cutanea tarda appears as blisters on sun-exposed areas or areas of trauma—usually on fingers and hands. Porphyria cutanea tarda responds to iron removal by taking blood (phlebotomy) and treatment of the hepatitis C.

Autoimmune Conditions. Case reports suggest that a number of autoimmune conditions may be associated with the hepatitis C virus or interferon treatment. These include idiopathic thrombocytopenic purpura (low platelet count), autoimmune chronic active hepatitis (inflammation in the liver due to your immune system), arthritis, Sjögren's syndrome (dry eyes and mouth), Raynaud's syndrome (blanching and numbness of fingers and toes), vasculitis (inflammation of small blood vessels), and polyarteritis nodosa (inflammation of large blood vessels, particularly in the abdomen, liver, and kidney).

Disorders that may flare on interferon therapy include hemolytic anemia (red cells break down), pericarditis/pleuritis (inflammation of the lining of the heart and lung), psoriasis, rheumatoid arthritis, and systemic lupus erythematosis.

Reading this list of what can go wrong with your liver anticipates the worst that can happen. Remember that more than two-thirds of the people who develop chronic hepatitis C do not progress to cirrhosis over 20 to 30 years. Nevertheless, it's important to know what the symptoms are, so you can report any changes promptly to your physician.

In the next chapters, we'll take a look at ways you can help your liver with healthy eating habits and stress-reduction techniques. I'll contribute a medical perspective, we'll hear from experts who specialize in these areas, and we'll listen to patients as they share their personal stories.

The beginning of health is to know the disease.

Miguel de Cervantes

References

1. Pablo Neruda. *Nuevas Odas Elementales.* Buenos Aires: Editorial Losada, p. 76–80.

2. "Sculpture in Spain Salutes the 'Silent, Unselfish' Liver," *Austin American-Statesman,* 28 June 1987:A2.

5

TAKING CARE OF YOURSELF NUTRITIONALLY

Guidelines for Healthy Nutrition in Liver Disease

At first, when I was still in shock over the diagnosis of chronic hepatitis C, I was too scared to try interferon. So I decided to do all I could with "natural" methods. I went to two dieticians who recommended a low-fat diet to take a load off my liver. They also advocated intravenous vitamin C and coffee enemas, which turned me off.

Then I saw a naturopath. He restricted my diet so much that I lost ten pounds. I never looked so good! But I still felt tired, so I consulted a nutritionist. She told me to keep a food journal, which made it possible for us to review my diet and my eating patterns.

I had been skimping on protein because I thought that would help my liver. Turns out that protein restriction is only for people in end-stage liver disease who are mentally confused. The nutritionist suggested I eat an appropriate amount of protein but divide it into smaller portions throughout the day.

Looking back, I can see what I was trying to do—control what I could in a world that suddenly seemed so out of control. I might not be able to stop the virus, but I could decide what I put into my body.

After a while, I found that all the junk food I used to love didn't taste so good anymore. It seems ironic to me now, but learning I was ill made me "healthier."

Hedy

MANY PEOPLE, when they discover they have hepatitis C, become interested in improving their general health through good nutrition. I encourage patients to learn how to eat in a healthier way, but to avoid crash diets and food fads that promise more than they can deliver.

Caution: Always check with your doctor before making major changes in your diet or taking over-the-counter supplements and vitamins. Some seemingly harmless substances can injure your liver.

In the early, noncirrhotic stages of hepatitis C, people can maintain normal nutrition if they eat a well-balanced diet. It's rare for a doctor to recommend supplements beyond one multivitamin a day. However, as the disease progresses, malnutrition and vitamin deficiencies may develop.

Nutritional therapy includes the following goals:

- to maintain the appropriate balance between the calories you take in and the calories your body requires
- to avoid malnutrition or deficiencies in specific nutrients
- to use appropriate supplementation when needed

In this chapter, I'll discuss some general nutritional concepts, what happens when liver disease affects your nutrition, and some specific deficiencies and their treatments:

- Nutritional Overview
  - Ideal Body Weight
  - Normal Diet
- Nutrition and the Liver
  - Carbohydrate Metabolism

Protein Metabolism

Fat Metabolism

Bile

Vitamins

• Nutritional Needs for Hepatitis C Patients without Cirrhosis

Caloric Requirements

Vitamin Supplements

Nutritional (Herbal) Therapies

Herbs Harmful to the Liver

Nutrition Tips from Patients

• Nutritional Needs for Hepatitis C Patients with Cirrhosis

Caloric Requirements

Protein Restriction

Vitamin Supplements

Mineral Supplements

Salt and Fluid Restriction

Nutritional Overview

The liver is your body's major digestive organ. When the liver receives nutrients from the intestines, it metabolizes★, packages, stores, and sends them to other organs where they are used for energy. Your liver's major nutritional jobs include:

• metabolizing carbohydrates, proteins, and fat for energy
• assimilating and storing vitamins
• manufacturing bile to aid in digestion and absorption of fats
• filtering and destroying toxins (including alcohol and drugs)

Ideal Body Weight. Most people worry about their weight with good reason. One in three American adults is overweight, a statistic that's up from one in four only a decade ago. With advanced liver disease, however, a major concern is the opposite problem, nutritional wasting.

What, then, should you weigh? We have no exact measure of ideal body weight because the "norm" is based on population statistics, cultural perceptions, and the influence of genetically and environmentally determined differences in metabolism. In short, there are no absolute rules, only working guidelines:

★Throughout this chapter we use the term "metabolism," which we define as the body processes, including a whole host of chemical reactions that are necessary to maintain function and sustain life.

- Men: 106 pounds for the first five feet, then add six pounds for every inch thereafter
- Women: 100 pounds for the first five feet, then add five pounds for every inch thereafter

Normal Diet. Food supplies us with carbohydrates, fats, and proteins that in turn supply energy. Energy is measured in calories. Carbohydrates and proteins provide approximately four calories per gram, and fat provides almost nine calories per gram—twice as much. People also need essential nutrients (such as certain vitamins, minerals, amino acids, and fatty acids) and other substances, such as fiber, from a variety of foods. Oranges, for example, are rich in vitamin C, bananas supply potassium, and a half-cup serving of cantaloupe contributes half of the daily requirement for beta-carotene.

> *I just read that lab tests at Cornell University show that natural chemicals in apples slow the growth rate of human liver cancer cells. The researchers said that they're not sure why, but it may be the antioxidants in fruits and vegetables—and it's best to eat a daily diet that includes five servings of a wide variety of fruits and vegetables.*
>
> *Ha! "An apple a day" really does keep the doctor away.*
>
> *Bonnie*

A normal, healthy diet contains the amounts of essential nutrients and calories you need to prevent either a nutritional deficiency or excess and provides the right balance of carbohydrate, fat, and protein. Many Americans, however, don't have good eating habits. According to the Healthy Eating Index of the U.S. Department of Agriculture (USDA) Center for Nutrition Policy and Promotion, only about 17 percent of people eat the recommended number of servings of fruit, and only about 31 percent eat the recommended number of servings of vegetables. In fact, diet-related health conditions (heart disease, stroke, cancer, and diabetes) "cost society about $250 billion annually in medical costs and lost productivity. Thirty to forty percent of deaths due to cancer can be prevented if people will choose a healthful diet and perform physical activity."[1]

What is a healthful diet? The USDA currently recommends a daily caloric intake of 30 to 40 calories per kilogram of body weight and the following dietary balance:

Food Guide Pyramid

A Guide to Daily Food Choices

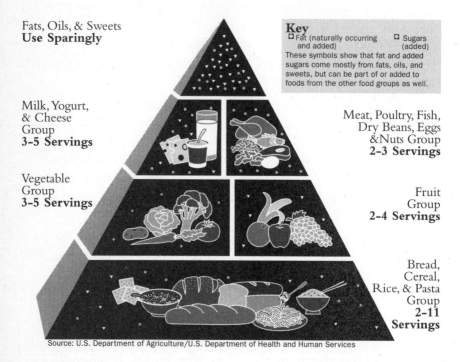

Fats, Oils, & Sweets
Use Sparingly

Key
□ Fat (naturally occurring   □ Sugars
and added)   (added)
These symbols show that fat and added
sugars come mostly from fats, oils, and
sweets, but can be part of or added to
foods from the other food groups as well.

Milk, Yogurt,
& Cheese
Group
3-5 Servings

Meat, Poultry, Fish,
Dry Beans, Eggs
&Nuts Group
2-3 Servings

Vegetable
Group
3-5 Servings

Fruit
Group
2-4 Servings

Bread,
Cereal,
Rice, & Pasta
Group
**2-11
Servings**

Source: U.S. Department of Agriculture/U.S. Department of Health and Human Services

Use the Food Guide Pyramid to help you eat better every day. . . the Dietary Guidelines way. Start with plenty of Breads, Cereals, Rice, and Pasta; Vegetables; and Fruits. And two to three servings from the Milk group and two to three servings from the Meat group.

Each of these food groups provides some, but not all, of the nutrients you need. No one food group is more important than another—for good health you need them all. Go easy on fats, oils, and sweets, the foods in the small tip of the Pyramid.

To order a copy of "The Food Guide Pyramid" booklet, send a $1.00 check or money order made out to the Superintendent of Documents to: Consumer Information Center, Department 1599-Y, Pueblo, Colorado 81009.

U.S. Department of Agriculture, Human Nutrition Information Service, August 1992, Leaflet No. 572

- 40 to 50 percent carbohydrate
- no more than 30 percent fat (less than 10 percent of calories from saturated fat)
- 1 to 1.5 grams of protein for each kilogram (2.2 lbs.) of body weight

For more information about healthy diets, I recommend you consult the Food Guide Pyramid published by the USDA. It graphically illustrates the importance of balance among different food groups in a daily eating pattern and suggests the number (depending on daily calorie intake desired) and size of daily servings. As you can see, you should choose a variety of grains (especially whole grains), fruits, and vegetables.

Pyramid serving sizes are not large. For example, one serving equals one-half cup of pasta; one cup of raw, leafy vegetables; one-half cup of other vegetables (cooked or chopped raw); one medium apple, banana, orange; one cup of milk or yoghurt; or two to three ounces of cooked lean meat, poultry, or fish.

The USDA recommendations include a range of servings from each of the five major food groups. People who consume about 1,600 calories a day should be guided by the smaller number; the larger number is for people who are very active and consume about 2,800 calories a day:

- Choose most of your daily foods from the bread, cereal, rice, and pasta group (6–11 servings), vegetable group (3–5 servings), and fruit group (2–4 servings).
- Choose moderate amounts of foods from the milk, yogurt, and cheese group (2–3 servings) and the meat, poultry, fish, dry beans, eggs, and nuts group (2–3 servings).
- Limit foods that provide few nutrients and are high in fat and sugar.
- In general, the USDA recommends a diet low in saturated fat and cholesterol and moderate in total fat. The new 2000 guidelines also urge you to choose appropriate beverages and foods in order to moderate your intake of sugars and salt.

Resource: For a free copy of *Dietary Guidelines for Americans,* call the USDA Center for Nutrition Policy and Promotion Publication Line: 202-606-8000 or write to 1120 20th St., NW, Suite 200, North Lobby, Washington, DC 20036. Website: usda.gov/cnpp

Resource: The American Dietetic Association's (ADA) National Referral Line (to find qualified dieticians in your area) is 1-800-366-1655. Helpful books: *Complete Food & Nutrition Guide* by Roberta Duyff and the ADA, and *Dieting for Dummies* by Jane Kirby and the ADA. Website: www.eatright.org

Resource: The American Institute for Cancer Research provides practical tips on good nutrition with its newsletter, pamphlets (ask for "The New American Plate" brochure), and a toll-free AICR Nutrition Hotline staffed by a registered dietician: Call 1-800-843-8114 and ask for Nutrition Information. Website: www.aicr.org

Resource: *Nutrition Action Newsletter* (Center for Science in the Public Interest). Website: www.cspinet.org

Resource: Track your "5 a day" minimum number of fruits and vegetables for a healthy diet and the average number of minutes you spend on daily exercise, along with recipes and tips for a healthy lifestyle at a website run by the National Cancer Institute and the CDC. Website: www.5aday.nci.nih.gov

Nutrition and the Liver

The liver is the major organ responsible for regulating and responding to your body's metabolic demands. Your liver must be functioning well to maintain normal metabolism of carbohydrates, fats, and protein; it is also responsible for processing and using several vitamins. This section deals with the role a healthy liver (and a healthy, well-balanced diet) plays in these nutritional processes.

Carbohydrate Metabolism. The most common sources of dietary carbohydrate are sugars, such as sucrose (table sugar), fructose (corn syrup), and lactose (milk sugar), and starches, such as breads, pasta, grains, cereals, fruits, vegetables, and potatoes. When you eat carbohydrates, specialized enzymes in the pancreas and gut process them to yield simple sugars (glucose, galactose, fructose, maltose).

These sugars are absorbed by intestinal lining cells, enter the portal circulation, and travel to the liver via the portal vein. During overnight fasting, blood sugar levels dip to a relatively low level, insulin secretion is suppressed, and blood insulin levels diminish. After a meal, blood sugar increases (stimulating the release of insulin from the pancreas), and insulin levels rise. Insulin, which rises in response to a meal, is the hormone that stimulates the liver to take in more glucose and to move the glucose into storage—mainly in the form of glycogen. The liver can then release glycogen to your muscles for energy during periods of fasting or exercise.

Although the liver can store considerable amounts of glycogen, it is the first energy source used during periods of prolonged fasting or caloric deprivation, and it can be depleted rapidly. After glycogen, the body taps other energy sources—including protein and fat.

Protein Metabolism. We take in dietary protein from dairy products, produce, and meats. Enzymes produced by the pancreas and intestine break down the protein into its amino acids and small peptides. The intestine rapidly absorbs the amino acids with specific transport systems within its lining cells and then delivers the amino acids to the liver via the portal vein.

When they reach the liver, they are used for energy or for making (synthesizing) new proteins. The newly synthesized proteins perform specific body functions (see Table 5A).

Fat Metabolism. In general, fats are neutral lipids (triglycerides), acidic lipids (fatty acids), and sterols (cholesterol, plant sterols). Triglycerides (dairy products, meats, oils, butter, margarine) are the most common type of dietary fat and represent a major source of energy. The liver is uniquely suited to regulate and process triglycerides.

Dietary triglyceride is digested in the intestine by lipase, an enzyme secreted by the pancreas in response to meals. Bile, secreted by the liver, makes the digested fat soluble and promotes its absorption. Absorbed fat is then repackaged and transported into blood, where the liver ultimately removes it from the circulation. Fat that reaches the liver is processed in three ways: (1) stored as fat droplets in liver cells, (2) metabolized as a source of energy, and (3) repackaged, secreted back into blood, and delivered to other cells in the body.

The liver is also intimately involved with the processing of dietary cholesterol and is the main source of newly synthesized cholesterol in the body. Liver disease may be associated with both high or low blood cholesterol levels. In general, as liver disease progresses in patients with hepatitis C, the blood level of cholesterol drops.

Bile. The liver produces and secretes a fluid (bile) that enters the intestine to aid in digestion and absorption. Bile is clear yellow to golden-brown and contains water, electrolytes (salts), cholesterol, bile salts (detergents), phospholipids, and proteins. Bile helps to activate enzymes secreted by the pancreas and is essential for the digestion and absorption of fat or fat-soluble vitamins.

Vitamins. The liver plays a role in several steps of vitamin metabolism. I'll describe only a few of those steps. Vitamins are either fat-solu-

TABLE 5A. SOME COMMON LIVER PROTEINS AND THEIR
FUNCTION IN THE HUMAN BODY

Protein	Function
Clotting Factors	
(II, V, VII, IX, and X)	Maintain normal clotting
Albumin	Maintain normal blood volume
Renin	Regulate blood pressure
Binding globulins	Regulate hormone action
Transferrin	Transport iron
Ferritin	Store iron
Retinol binding protein	Transport Vitamin A to the eye
LDL receptor	Remove Cholesterol from the blood
P-450 proteins	Metabolize drugs, chemicals, toxins

ble (vitamins A, D, E, and K) or water-soluble (vitamin C and the B-complex vitamins).

Patients with advanced liver disease may become deficient in water-soluble vitamins, but this is usually due to inadequate nutrition and poor food intake. Vitamin B12 storage usually far exceeds the body's requirements; deficiencies rarely occur due to liver disease or liver failure. When dietary intake drops, however, thiamine and folate commonly become deficient. Oral supplementation is usually all that you need to restore thiamine and folate stores to the normal range.

Fat-soluble vitamins require not only adequate dietary intake but also good digestion and absorption by the body. That's why normal production of bile is essential. Bile in the gut is required for the absorption of fat-soluble vitamins into the body because these vitamins are relatively insoluble in water. Bile acts as a detergent, breaking down and dissolving these vitamins so they may be properly absorbed.

If bile production is poor, oral supplementation of vitamins A, D, E, and K may not be sufficient to restore vitamin levels to normal. The use of a detergent-like solution of liquid vitamin E (TPGS) improves the absorption of vitamin E in patients with advanced liver disease. The same solution may also improve the absorption of vitamins A, D, and K if the latter are taken simultaneously with the liquid vitamin E.

Nutritional Needs for Hepatitis C Patients Who Don't Have Cirrhosis

Caloric Requirements. In general, the noncirrhotic patient with hepatitis C has caloric needs similar to those of noninfected people of the same age and gender. For this reason we recommend the following:

- no salt restriction
- no protein restriction
- 30 to 40 calories per kilogram intake per day
- one multivitamin per day

Patients who drink excessive amounts of alcohol should stop drinking altogether. They may also need supplementation with thiamine and folate.

Patients often proudly tell me that they are restricting their protein intake to "help" their livers. I'd like to emphasize that moderate amounts of protein (as recommended by the Food Pyramid) should be a normal part of your diet. If you are concerned about fat content, choose low-fat sources of protein. Protein restriction is recommended only for patients with cirrhosis who have encephalopathy (mental confusion).

Common questions I'm asked are, "Will dietary fat harm my liver? Should I avoid fat? Can I digest fat?" Dietary fat (triglycerides) undergoes complex processing (see Chapter 4). In the setting of liver disease, fat may accumulate in the liver. However, dietary fat intake does not correlate with the degree of fatty accumulation. Nonetheless, liver fat (steatosis) may promote liver injury and fibrosis in patients with viral hepatitis. Therefore, we do recommend a diet relatively low in fat, particularly saturated fat.

On the other hand, viral hepatitis by itself does not alter fat digestion or absorption from the gut. Only patients with advanced liver disease (cirrhosis) with jaundice have altered fat digestion and absorption. Jaundice in the setting of cirrhosis indicates severe impairment of processing and secretion of bile. Reduced bile concentration in the gut limits fat digestion and absorption.

Vitamin Supplements. In general, noncirrhotic patients with hepatitis C do not require any additional vitamin supplementation other than that noted above. One concern is that if bile production drops, the patient may become deficient in fat-soluble vitamins during the course of hepatitis C infection. This deficiency rarely develops during the early stages of hepatitis C, but it may be fairly prevalent at later, cirrhotic stages of the disease. When detected, deficiencies of fat-soluble vitamins should be corrected by administering proper doses of the compounds.

I am frequently asked, "Is it okay to take iron?" The answer goes beyond a simple yes or no. Women who are actively ovulating tend to lose iron through menstruation. Some of these women may develop iron deficiency and anemia, and they may actually benefit from iron. Men and non-ovulatory or post-menopausal women typically are not iron-deficient, and supplementation is not necessary. In fact, inappropriate supplementation with iron-loaded vitamins may be harmful in patients with liver disease.

One theory of the development of liver disease is that oxidant stress promotes liver cell injury and also stimulates specialized cells in the liver (stellate cells) to produce the main fibrosis protein, collagen. Iron is a catalyst for oxidant injury by promoting formation of "free radicals" that can initiate injury and fibrosis.

Supplemental vitamin C may be of potential benefit because it has antioxidant properties. However, vitamin C may promote iron absorption and lead to excessive accumulation of iron in the liver. The latter effect could actually increase oxidant injury. A reasonable, middle-ground approach is to take in the daily FDA-recommended amount of vitamin C and to avoid excessive supplementation.

Nutritional (Herbal) Therapies. According to the *Nutrition Business Journal,* supplements were a $15.4 billion dollar industry in 1999.[2] Patients with viral hepatitis have used a number of "nutritional supplements," such as echinaceae, pycnogenol, dandelion root, silymarin (milk thistle), and a wide array of herbal remedies. Most of these have not been studied in controlled trials and, thus, are unproved therapies. Silymarin has been studied but has not demonstrated clear benefit.

Despite the lack of supporting data, the use of these therapies has gained widespread acceptance among patients with hepatitis C. Several factors seem to account for this phenomenon: a history of lack of effective therapies for liver disease in general; incompletely effective treatment for hepatitis C; a general attitude that, "It can't hurt me, and maybe it'll help"; and the relatively mild and slowly progressive nature of hepatitis C.

Herbs have been used to treat illness since time began. In fact, many modern pharmaceuticals were discovered in natural sources. Aspirin originally came from the bark of the white willow tree. Cyclosporin, the miracle drug that suppresses the immune system and makes liver transplants possible, was found in a fungus growing in the soil of a plateau in southern Norway.

I have no doubt that future controlled studies of herbs for liver disease will result in useful treatments. Saw palmetto, for example, has been studied in a controlled trial by New York University researchers and found effective in certain doses for prostrate conditions. Some "natural" substances are ineffective, and others may be as powerful as approved Western medicines. However, until we have proof of effectiveness and safety, I cannot endorse or recommend that patients undergo nutritional therapies.

Quality control of potency and contaminants is another problem. In 1998, California investigators found that "nearly one-third of 260 imported Asian herbals were either spiked with drugs not listed on the label or contained lead, arsenic or mercury."[3]

In addition, herbs can interact with other medications you may be taking. For example, St. John's wort, a popular herbal antidepressant, recently has been found to decrease levels of life-sustaining cyclosporine in heart transplant patients.[4]

I do not recommend using herbs, but if you are interested in them, become informed. And remember that it is vitally important to tell your doctor if you are taking any nutritional supplement.

Under current laws, herbs classified as food or dietary supplements are exempt from regulations governing quality control and proof of effectiveness. Often, people will take the recommendations of the clerk who sells the supplements.

> *I went to a health food store and asked them to give me anything that would help my liver. I got coltsfoot, comfrey, petasites, chaparral, and yohimbe.*
>
> *My enzymes shot up to 800. When the doctor asked me if I was taking anything new, I brought in the bottles and learned that these herbs were best avoided because they may be toxic for the liver. I stopped taking them, and my enzymes went back down. I never thought anything "natural" could harm me.*
>
> *Harold*

Why isn't more research done on herbs? In 1978, the German government set up Commission E. The agency doesn't conduct research, but it does review studies and other evidence of safety and effectiveness, including anecdotal reports, and publishes its findings. Congress responded to public interest and increased funding for the National Institutes of Health (NIH) Center for Complementary and Alternative Medicine/Office of Alternative Medicine from $50 million for fiscal year 1999 to $68.7 million for fiscal year 2000. The largest portion of the funding goes to herbal product research.

In 1994 Congress passed the Dietary Supplement Health and Education Act (DSHEA) that gave dietary supplement manufacturers the freedom to market more products. The Food and Drug Administration (FDA) must review clinical studies of drugs to determine effectiveness, safety, dosages, and possible interactions with other substances. Under DSHEA, however, the FDA does not authorize or test dietary supplements, and manufacturers do not need the agency's approval of ingredients and products before marketing.

Herbs Harmful to the Liver. After a dietary supplement is on the market, the FDA has the responsibility for showing that it is unsafe before it can take action to restrict use. In June 1997 the FDA proposed to limit the amount of ephedrine alkaloids in dietary supplements (marketed as ephedra, Ma Huang, Chinese ephedra, and epitonin, for example) and to provide warnings to consumers about hazards (including hepatitis) associated with use of these substances.[5]

In 1993 the FDA named before a Senate committee other supplements as possible hazards associated with illness and injuries to the liver. The list includes Chaparral, Comfrey, Germander, vitamin A (in doses of 25,000 or more International Units a day), and niacin (in slow-release doses of 500 mg. or more a day or immediate-release doses of 750 mg. or more a day).

Here's a list I give to my patients of herbs that have been documented to cause liver problems ranging from hepatitis to liver failure: Atractylis Gummifera, Azadirachza indica, Berberis vulgaris, Calliepsis laureola, Cassia angustifolia (Senna), Crotaiaria, Corydalis, Hedeoma pulegoides, Heliotropium, Larrea tridentata (Chaparral bush, Creosote bush, Greasewood), Lycopodium serratum (Jin Bu Huan), Mentha pulegoides, Sassafras albidum (Sassafras), Scuteileria (Skullcap), Stephania, Symphytum officinale (Comfrey), Teucrium chamaedrys [Germander (mint family)], Tussilago farfara (Peppermint), Valeriana officinalis

(Valerian, Asfetida, Hops, Gentian), Viscum alba [Mistletoe, Margosa oil, Mate tea, Gordolobo yerba tea, Pennyroyal (squawmint) oil];[6] Senecio, Heliotropium, Chelidonum majus (greater celandine), and "a variety of Chinese herbal mixtures (artemisia, hare's ear, chrysanthemum, plantago seed, gardinia, red peony root, etc.").[7]

In my opinion, if you have a chronic liver disease, such as hepatitis C, you should avoid herbs that have not been tested in controlled studies, especially if you are being treated with interferon. Any substance, such as herbs or over-the-counter medications, may interact with drugs you are taking. Always discuss medicines and herbs with your physician.

Resource: Food and Drug Administration, Office of Consumer Affairs, HFE-88, Rockville, MD 20857. Consumer Food Information Line (Center for Food Safety and Applied Nutrition Outreach and Information Center): 1-800-FDA-4010 (in Washington, D.C., call 202-205-4314). FDA Website: www.cfsan.fda.gov/~dms/supplmnt.html

Resources: Contact the National Institutes of Health (NIH) National Center for Complementary and Alternative Medicine (NCCAM)/Office of Alternative Medicine Clearinghouse at 1-888-644-6226. Website: http://altmed.od.nih.gov

Access the NCCAM website with links to thousands of scientific citations related to complementary and alternative medicine. Website: http://nccam.nih.gov

Access the NIH Office of Dietary Supplements website for more information on nutritional supplements. Website: http://dietary-supplements.info.nih.gov/

Resource: The National Digestive Disease Information Clearinghouse (NDDIC) offers a brochure, "Harmful Effects of Medicines on the Adult Digestive System," which describes some over-the-counter and prescription drugs that may affect the liver. Call 301-654-3810. Website: www.niddk.nih.gov

Resource: Tyler, Varro E. *The Honest Herbal: A Sensible Guide to the Use of Herbs and Related Remedies.* New York: Pharmaceutical Products Press. 1993.

Resource: Gruenwald, Joerg, Thomas Brendler, Christof Jaenicke. *PDR® for Herbal Medicines.* Montvale: Medical Economics. 2000.

Nutrition Tips from Patients. People with hepatitis C who are interested in nutrition find many ways to work toward healthier eating habits. Here are some of their suggestions:

I think you're crazy if you have hepatitis C and you drink alcohol. It's like taking poison.

I try to be kind to my liver. I've switched to eating more complex carbohydrates, like veggies, fruits, whole grains. If Olympic athletes train on complex carbs for energy, I guess it's good for me, too.

I've given up caffeine. I figure it can't do my liver any good. So every morning I have hot water with a bit of fresh lemon in it. It was hard to switch at first, but I'm used to it now.

I don't tolerate fats as well as I did. I can't handle the beans, chili, and tortillas I used to eat—too fatty and salty. I can't handle fried foods at all. When I cook at home, I use mostly olive oil—sometimes canola oil.

Eating small meals several times a day works better for me than eating a few large meals because I don't have much appetite. I also keep unsalted nuts in the car, in case I need a quick protein snack.

Hot oatmeal tastes good on a cold morning. To add a little protein, I sprinkle some unsalted nuts on top. Also—to avoid using too much sugar, I add just a little bit of maple syrup. It's sugar, too, but a little goes a long way.

I used to drink 2 percent milk. Turns out that it is not low in fat. In fact, 35 percent of its calories comes from fat. So I switched to skim milk. Now I like it just as well, and it has almost no fat in it.

I used to drink lots of soda, too, until I looked at the labels—lots of sugar and salt and preservatives. I stopped all soda about a year ago. The other day I took a taste of a friend's drink and almost spit it out. My taste buds have changed.

You should see my new juicer. I'm a little intimidated by it, but I made the sweetest, freshest tasting carrot juice today. I've also heard that a carrot, beet, and cucumber combo is good, too. I figured I'd drink some of my veggies.

A lot is attitude. If you think of a healthy, low-fat diet as a pleasure—not a burden—you can get into it. I take the time to shop in a really pleasant supermarket or health food store, and I try to add new fruits and vegetables to my meals or snacks.

I try to sit down and not eat on the run. My biggest problem is that I have to eat out a lot for business, but I've learned to order fish and rice more often.

Nutritional Needs for Hepatitis C Patients with Cirrhosis

Caloric Requirements. In general, the patient with early-stage or compensated cirrhosis still requires 30 to 40 calories per kilogram a day. You may need to alter your dietary habits to take in this number of calories, because as hepatitis C progresses to cirrhosis, you may begin to experience loss of appetite, increasing fatigue, reduction in physical activity, and alteration of your sleep-wake pattern. People commonly complain of loss of exercise tolerance ("I'm just too pooped out to get my work done"). In addition, these changes often precipitate a sense of despondency, anxiety, or depression. It helps to develop both a pattern of meals that allows you to use your diet for maximum energy and a rest pattern that reduces prolonged periods of physical activity.

No nutritional prescription is right for every patient. You need to address your specific nutritional needs with your physician. In my experience, patients with hepatitis C who develop compensated cirrhosis benefit by more frequent, smaller volume meals. Instead of one or two large meals, divide the equivalent amount of calories into four smaller meals. In addition, supplementation with one or two tablets of multivitamins is generally indicated, although the overall benefit is unclear. Despite this change in dietary habit, fatigue often persists. People benefit from "rest periods," usually 30 minutes or an hour in the mid-afternoon.

Caution: Please understand that advanced cirrhosis is associated with severe impairment of liver function and that specific dietary modifications may be necessary and could alter the general guidelines noted above. Your doctor may recommend a consultation with a dietician or provide you with a specific nutritional prescription.

Protein Restriction. It is important that the patient with cirrhosis take in enough protein to avoid excessive muscle wasting and energy depletion. However, if encephalopathy develops, a doctor might prescribe a "protein-restricted" diet.

Encephalopathy is the alteration or cloudiness of mental function. When the condition is severe, the patient becomes disoriented, confused, combative, or even comatose. Encephalopathy may also cause altered sleep-wake patterns, altered personality, and lack of motor coordination.

One factor contributing to these symptoms is dietary protein intake, so patients with any of the above symptoms may be placed on protein restrictions. This diet is usually not zero protein, but a reduced level of 20 to 60 grams per day. Often, the physician will use other treatments in conjunction with this diet, such as lactulose or neomycin.

> *While I was waiting for my liver transplant, I'd get in the car and forget if I was leaving or coming. If you've got too much protein, it can cause you to fall asleep at the intersection. The doctor told me to stop driving and put me on a protein-restricted diet. I watch the amount I take in, and if I feel too tired, I cut back. It took lots of modification to eat more vegetables. I eat them like medicine, but I'm getting better at it.*
>
> *I'm from South Dakota. I was raised on meat and potatoes. In fact, my parents joke that I was 16 before I found out that gravy wasn't a beverage!*
>
> *Bill*

Vitamin Supplements. Most people with hepatitis C, even those with cirrhosis, have adequate intake and storage of water-soluble vitamins (C, B complex). To be sure, I recommend the addition of two tablets of multivitamins each day (one in the morning and one in the evening).

Patients who excessively use or abuse alcohol risk becoming deficient in these vitamins, particularly thiamine and folate, and they may benefit from taking supplements. As I have emphasized before, the hepatitis C patient should avoid alcohol. Those who avoid alcohol probably won't require either supplement.

There are few data on the overall extent of vitamin deficiencies in patients with hepatitis C. However, as part of our evaluation of cirrhotic patients for liver transplantation, we assessed the plasma levels of certain vitamins and found that approximately 20 percent of hepatitis C patients were deficient in vitamin A, vitamin D (25-OH), and vitamin E. Although few patients had symptoms that could be attributed to these deficiencies, it seems reasonable to monitor patients' vitamin levels as cirrhosis progresses and give supplements to those with low levels.

Mineral Supplements. Patients with cirrhosis may experience deficiencies in three minerals: calcium, magnesium, and zinc. Calcium deficiency may be related to a lack of vitamin D, poor nutrition, or malabsorption. Correcting the underlying abnormality may be all that is required to restore calcium balance. However, bone thinning may occur even without these specific problems, so I recommend 0.5 to 1.0 grams of calcium each day. Calcium may be taken in the form of dairy products or therapeutic supplements. When the patient can't take in enough dairy products because of protein, salt, or fluid restrictions (see next section), supplements are used.

Magnesium deficiency may occur due to inadequate dietary intake. However, it occurs more often when patients take diuretics to treat fluid retention because their kidneys flush out the magnesium as waste. Symptoms of magnesium deficiency include muscle cramps, fatigue, weakness, nausea, and vomiting. Often, it's not possible to modify or discontinue diuretics in cirrhotic patients, so magnesium supplementation (500 mg. magnesium gluconate three times a day) may be required.

Zinc deficiency may cause the loss of the senses of smell and taste. Patients with these symptoms may benefit from supplementation with zinc sulfate (220 mg. three times a day).

Salt and Fluid Restriction. Cirrhosis disturbs the regulation of body salt and water. Severe liver disease generates neural and hormonal signals to the kidney that cause the kidney to retain both salt and water. The salt acts like a sponge. As a result, fluid accumulates in certain tissues and body spaces, such as the ankles (peripheral edema), abdomen (ascites), and chest (pleural effusion).

TABLE 5B. 2–GRAM SALT DIET SAMPLE MENU*

Breakfast (352–765 mg)
1–2 pieces toast (150–400 mg)
1–2 tsp. margarine (50 mg)
1 Tbs. orange marmalade
1 boiled egg (62 mg)
    or 1 fried egg (162 mg)
1 C cooked cereal with little or no salt (1 mg)
½–1 C milk (60–120 mg)
6 oz. brewed coffee (4 mg)/tea (5 mg)/herbal tea (2 mg)
1 C cantaloupe (14 mg) or strawberries (2 mg)
1 C orange juice (2 mg)

Lunch (503–611 mg)
3.5 oz. salmon patty (96 mg)
1 slice tomato (½ mg) and ½ C lettuce (1 mg)
1 oz. potato chips (about 10 chips) (170 mg)
1 C fresh grapes (2 mg)
1 C apple juice (7 mg)
1 carrot (25 mg) and 1 stalk of celery (3.5 mg)
1 piece angel food cake [161 mg (homemade); approx. 270 mg
    (packaged mix)]
8 oz. ice tea (5 mg) with lemon (less than 1 mg)

Dinner (431–601 mg)
3.5 oz. roast beef (63–73 mg) au jus with no added salt
    (if packaged gravy mix, 2 oz. = approx. 160 mg)
1 baked potato (16 mg)
1 tbsp. sour cream (6mg)/marge (100 mg)
½ C frozen green beans (3 mg)
1½ C tossed fresh salad (5 mg) with salt-free salad dressing
1 piece apple (181 mg) with ½ C vanilla ice cream (53 mg)
6 oz. coffee (4 mg)

*   *Sodium levels generally refer to fresh homemade items, are approximate,
    and vary with brand names of products used. Fast, pre-packaged, or canned
    foods usually contain much higher levels of sodium.*

The dietician restricted me to 2,000 milligrams of sodium a day. That's one teaspoon! I try, but I really like salt. If I don't watch carefully, though—say I eat some broth, and it has salt in it—I pick up extra water. It takes days to flush it out.

I can get 11 to 14 pounds of fluid out every few days. Once I had 30 pounds of water on me. I had a belly like a pregnant rhino.

My wife says if I wouldn't cover everything with "white death," I'd do a lot better.

Randy

Treatment of fluid retention always requires dietary salt restriction, often requires diuretics (medicines that block the kidney and cause increased urination of salt and water), and sometimes requires fluid restriction. Patients need to understand that the major driving force behind the accumulation of fluid is the excessive retention of salt. Diuretics work because they cause the kidney to lose salt. If you take in too much salt in your diet, you'll cause more fluid to accumulate in your body. In other words, you can override the effects of the diuretics, and patients on diuretics can actually retain fluid if they don't comply with a salt-restricted diet.

The usual salt restriction is two grams per day (see Table 5B). Commonly used diuretics are Aldactone® (spironolactone), Midamor® (amiloride), Lasix® (furosemide), HCTZ® (hydrochlorothiazide), and Zaroxylyn® (metolozone). Aldactone® and Midamor® conserve potassium, while Lasix®, HCTZ®, and Zaroxylyn® waste potassium. Most of the time, a doctor will prescribe the two types of diuretics together to minimize any changes in blood potassium levels. Occasionally, potassium supplements are used to keep blood potassium in the normal range.

The physician usually orders fluid restriction only for edematous (swollen with fluid) patients with low levels of sodium in their blood. Fluid restriction means restriction of all fluids: water, tea, coffee, milk, etc. Patients with severe symptomatic low blood sodium may find it necessary to restrict their fluid intake to less than one quart a day.

Caution: Always consult with your physician regarding use of diuretics (doses and frequency) or dietary restrictions on salt or fluid intake. It is potentially dangerous to self-medicate or introduce dietary restrictions without physician consultation.

He who keeps on eating after his stomach is full
digs his grave with his teeth.

Turkish proverb

References

1. "Q and A's on Dietary Guidelines for Americans, 2000." 3 June 2000, *Center for Nutrition Policy and Promotion.* 1 Sept. 2000 <www.usda.gov/cnpp/Pubs/DG2000/Qa5-2.pdf.>

2. "NBJ's Fifth Annual Overview of the Nutrition Industry," *Nutrition Business Journal* Vol. V No. 7/8 2000:1.

3. Guy Gugliotta, "Supplements Aren't So Healthy," *Denver Post* March 19, 2000: 5A.

4. T.H. Breidenbach, M.W. Hoffman, T.H. Becker, H. Schlitt, J. Klempnauer. "Drug Interaction of St. John's Wort with Cyclosporine." *Lancet.* 27 May 2000; 355:1912.

5. Paula Kurtzweil, "An FDA Guide to Dietary Supplements," *FDA Consumer* Sept.-Oct. 1998:29.

6. D. Larrey, G.P. Pageaux. "Hepatotoxicity of Herbal Remedies and Mushrooms." *Seminars in Liver Disease.* 1995; 15:183-188.

7. D. Schuppan, J.D. Jia, B. Brinkhaus, E.G. Hahn. "Herbal Products for Liver Diseases: A Therapeutic Challenge for the New Millennium." *Hepatology.* 1999; 30:1100.

6

TAKING CARE OF YOURSELF EMOTIONALLY

Emotional Challenges of Chronic Illness

As a person with hepatitis C, I live with the emotional highs and lows of this disease. Every blood test and biopsy report shakes me up. Every time I get tired and can't get through a job that I used to do easily, I get angry and discouraged. It's a struggle not to get obsessed with my health.

Some days, I get mad when my friends act too protective, and other times I get mad when they leave me alone. It's hard to shake off the sadness. And then there are those glorious moments—a crisp fall day, a family dinner—when life is a gift that's unbearably beautiful.

Hedy

IN THIS CHAPTER, Dr. Everson and I draw on the expertise of mental health professionals who work with hepatitis C patients. We also present the experiences of the patients themselves. Who else really understands?

Here are the topics we'll cover:

• The Emotional Challenge
• Phase 1: Diagnosis
• Special Problems with a Diagnosis of Hepatitis C
• Phase 2: Impact (Attitudes and Expectations)
• Phase 3: Reorganization
• Healing vs. Curing
• Warning Signs of Depression
• Understanding your Family and Friends (Family Systems)
    Boundaries
• Tools for Wellness: Some Practical Suggestions
    Medical Care and Psychological Help
    Exercise and Nutrition
    Feeling Useful/Having Fun
    Exploring Your Creative and Spiritual Sides

The Emotional Challenge

Hepatitis C may be the biggest emotional challenge you'll ever face. How do you deal with chronic disease without letting it take over your life?

"The goal is balance," says Meredith Pate-Willig, a licensed clinical social worker. Ms. Pate-Willig facilitates support groups for Denver's Qualife, an organization that seeks to enrich the quality of life for people facing life-challenging illness.

How do you achieve balance and a "wellness lifestyle?" "There's no shortcut through normal, natural cycles of grief," says Pate-Willig. "Grieving is nature's way of helping us adapt to new information about our illness."

Too often, we're hard on ourselves as we grieve. In a world of instant cereal and microwave popcorn, we think we should be grieving faster, better. The truth is, each one of us goes through the process in our own time frame and in our own way—and the healing ingredient is kindness. Be patient with yourself. You will work it through, and you will come out of the crisis with a stronger sense of who you are.

According to Pate-Willig, it's helpful to think of these spiraling cycles of grief in three phases: diagnosis, impact, and reorganization.

Phase 1: Diagnosis

Diagnosis plunges you into a state of disbelief or shock.

> *I didn't realize it then, but it was the day my life changed forever. I was numb. I didn't even know that I was feeling shock and grief at what I had lost—my sense of health. When I walked out to the parking lot, the sun was still shining, but everything looked different. It felt unreal.*
>
> *Dave*

If you lose your sense of yourself as a healthy person, and you struggle or rebel against becoming a patient, how do you adjust? Some patients develop a sense of grief. Grieving is one way we work through loss, whether it's loss of our old selves ("I used to cook big family dinners. Now I'm too tired.") or loss of our dreams ("Will I ever marry now? Know my grandchildren? Launch a new business?"). According to Pate-Willig, "Grieving is normal—even necessary. It's the bridge between what was to what is. If you don't go across that bridge, you may face a continuing struggle."

In this first phase of diagnosis, you need your family and support system to pull together to help you adjust:

1. The diagnosis may make you feel uncomfortable or leave you with a numbing sense of shock and loss. You should understand that this response is normal.
2. Everyone needs psychological and social support—not just the person with hepatitis C. Other family members may be affected by the diagnosis. When one part of a system changes, everything in the system reacts in a "ripple" effect.

> *When I was first diagnosed, I went numb. The first person I told was my best friend. She broke down—a flood of tears. I was horrified to find that my inner reaction was rage. I wanted to yell, "Hey, just a minute. I'm the one with the problem here!"*
>
> *Thank goodness, I didn't say anything out loud, but I was mad until I realized that she had her own grief about losing me, her best friend, as she's always known me. Her world was shaken up, too.*

All I wanted, all I ever really want even now, is for someone to put an arm around me and say, "I'm here. I know this is hard. I care about you."

Estelle

People may not respond to you in the way that you anticipate or expect. You may process the information fast while family members take longer, or the reverse. How fast or how slowly people absorb the news affects the dynamics in a marriage or friendship—leaving everyone with the unconscious feeling that somehow the rules changed. In fact, just identifying these changes takes a while.

Sometimes, the patient or support system refuses to accept the new reality. "Denial," says Pate-Willig, "is a misunderstood defense. When it acts as a circuit-breaker, it keeps your system from overloading. That can be healthy. Denial becomes unhealthy when it keeps you from finding appropriate medical treatment."

Special Problems with a Diagnosis of Hepatitis C

Dealing with a diagnosis of any chronic illness is difficult, but patients with hepatitis C have special issues:

Feeling Low. You may be experiencing fatigue, low energy, loss of ability to concentrate, and a sense of inadequacy in doing daily tasks. These symptoms may make you more emotionally vulnerable and susceptible to periods of depression. Be sure to tell your doctor if you feel seriously depressed.

Feeling Contaminated. Although the virus is transmitted only by blood-to-blood contact, you may have questions and fears about who will avoid you. How will your friends or boss react? What do you tell your dentist?

I can't believe this guy at work. I left a can of pop on the table for a minute, and he drank it by mistake. He freaked out when he found out it was mine. Now he won't even talk to me if he can help it. When he passes my desk, he won't even look me in the eye!

Bonnie

How You Got Infected. When you try to figure out how this happened to you, your answer may affect how you deal with your diagnosis: (1) If you can point to a blood transfusion, you don't feel responsible for your illness; (2) if you've injected drugs, whether it was a minor episode or you're still involved, you have to process the painful idea that you did this to yourself; (3) people who don't know how they got infected may never figure it out, and that uncertainty creates its own dilemmas.

Looking Good. Strange as it sounds, people often have trouble offering comfort to someone who doesn't have a visible wound. In the early and middle stages of infection, you may suffer silent symptoms, such as fatigue and joint pains. Unfortunately, many people (including yourself) may have a hard time believing you're ill. Unless you explain the nature of hepatitis C, you may not get the support you need.

> *For years before I was diagnosed, I dealt with an energy level that seemed to be going downhill. I stopped playing tennis because I couldn't run fast enough to get to the ball. I had to give up biking when my knees ached so bad.*
>
> *Now I just learned I have hepatitis C, but my wife doesn't listen. "You look fine," she says. "You're just getting older."*
>
> *George*

Fluctuating Nature of Hepatitis C. Who knows why a person's PCR assay shows a low viral load one month but a sky-high count the next? The fluctuating course of hepatitis C sometimes gives the patient the feeling of walking on shifting sand, never knowing what each day will bring.

Lack of Information. Uncertainty due to lack of information is a huge stressor. You have no way to answer the questions, "What am I dealing with, and how will it affect my life?" What facts your doctor offers you about your stage of illness, therefore, have a big influence on how you deal with the diagnosis.

What Can You Do to Help Yourself? "Be patient with yourself," says Pate-Willig. "Accept that this is a difficult time, and try not to beat yourself up for being normal, human."

The results of my second biopsy sent me into a tailspin. My liver was worse! It was like going back to the first day I was told I had hepatitis C. For days and weeks I struggled to control panic attacks and crying jags. I couldn't get on top of it.

Finally, a friend with hepatitis C told me not to stuff the pain and sadness. "The only thing that works for me," she said, "is to feel it all the way."

When I gave myself time to feel whatever it was—no matter how painful—I was able to move on with the rest of my day. I didn't get stuck.

Lani

"Remember to be kind to yourself. Patience, patience, and more patience. That's the key," says Pate-Willig. "Expect to feel emotional cycles, ups and downs, each time the activity of your disease changes or you experience a new symptom."

Phase 2: Impact (Attitudes and Expectations)

In Phase 1, the task for you and your support system is to pull together to confront and understand the new diagnosis. In the second phase, the question becomes, "How do we function now that we know that hepatitis C is a chronic condition? How do we gear up for the long haul?" It's a time of changing attitudes and expectations as you explore your options.

The challenge is how to connect with friends and family and still maintain the autonomy and space you need. Your questions may vary from large ("I'm a single parent with no one to care for me. Should I go back to my mom and dad's house or keep my own apartment?") to small ("My husband had a transplant. Should I play in my Thursday night bowling league or stay home with him?").

Families often have unspoken rules and myths about illness. Perhaps the message you got was, "Keep a stiff upper lip and don't show you're scared." Or maybe you grew up in a home where a cold meant deluxe pampering. What happens if you break these rules?

I finally told my older brother how scared and panicky I felt. It turned out that my brother had a friend who also had hepatitis C. "He doesn't make any big deal," my brother said. "In fact, he won't even discuss it. He believes in a positive outlook."

Compared to my brother's friend, I was a big complainer. Of course, that was my secret fear all along—being the family wimp.

Melissa

Phase 3: Reorganization

As you move into Phase 3, you and your family begin to reorganize around the new reality. A sense of acceptance emerges, and you start to answer these questions: Who am I now? How am I going to make my life work?

At some point, things settle down. Perhaps you come to terms with a reduced energy level, make dietary changes, decide on a treatment plan.

It got to be too much for me. I couldn't even cope with a full work day. Cassie and I had planned a mountain climbing vacation in the Rockies, but we decided to spend a week at a bed-and-breakfast with a mountain view instead. Finally, I had to accept reality.

Jim

Anything that tips the precarious balancing act shakes the system. If you start interferon treatment, you and your family and friends may need to organize around the treatment. Suppose you decide to plan a nap each day, while someone else assumes your chores. What most people don't realize is that *any* change, positive or negative, alters the system. So, paradoxically, you may need to reorganize after you have finished interferon treatment. For example, you may still feel the need for a daily nap, but the people around you may now disapprove.

The cycle of confronting the diagnosis, feeling its impact, and reorganizing yourself to deal with hepatitis C may recur with each piece of health news. If hepatitis C moves into advanced liver disease and a possible transplant, the concept of death may come to the forefront.

"The first big breakthrough for most people is the realization of how physically fragile we humans are," says Pate-Willig. "It's a difficult task to process, reprioritize, accept your mortality, and—at the same time—plan for post-transplant living."

Healing vs. Curing

"We are all desperate for curing," says Pate-Willig, "but a physical cure may be years away. We need to shift to healing—a balance and wholeness of mind, body, and spirit.

"As we become more aware of our emotional responses, we learn how healthy it is to *lean* into the grief process and accept it. We learn how to tap into resources that can help, such as dietary changes and relaxation techniques. The goal is to come out of each cycle at a higher level, to feel better about ourselves, and to see more flexibility in ourselves and others as we learn how to cope."

Grief can be the great healer. Grief is to the psyche and the spirit what the physical process is to the healing of a wound.

So, you say, "That sounds great. But how do I grieve?"

"Talk about what's happening to you," says Pate-Willig. Talk to a friend, a support group, a journal. Get on the Internet. Help yourself by re-evaluating your feelings each time you tell and retell your story. As you do this, you fit your new self into your old idea of yourself.

"The Chinese symbol for crisis is both danger and opportunity. Chronic illness can give us the opportunity to become deeper, broader, more flexible, and to find meaning in our lives."

Warning Signs of Depression

While grieving and depression are normal, sustained depression is not. Fortunately, there are many ways to treat depression with medications and "talk" therapy, so it's important to tell your doctor, advises Robert House, M.D., Director of Residency Training and the Department of Psychiatric Consultation Liaison Service for the University of Colorado Health Sciences Center.

What are the signs of depression? According to Dr. House, be on the alert for some of these symptoms, if they are *changes* from your normal behavior pattern:

- low energy, fatigue, lack of interest in your usual activities
- withdrawn and/or irritable behavior

- sleep disturbances that show a change in your routine pattern (such as sleeping less or more, waking up a lot, or waking earlier or later than usual, not rested and ready to begin the day)
- significant weight loss over a short period of time
- loss of appetite, food doesn't taste good
- tearfulness, breaking into tears for no apparent reason, "out of the blue"
- forming and talking about ideas of suicide, or a sense that life is not worth living
- feeling of hopelessness, helplessness that things won't get better
- reluctance to resume activities of daily living after a transplant (such as not getting along with your family, if you've always done so before; not resuming sexual relations with your spouse after a reasonable length of time; not dating, if single; isolating yourself from others).

Understanding Your Family and Friends (Family Systems)

Chronic illness is a family illness. When one member of a family becomes sick, it affects everyone. Normally, a family stays in balance with its own set of unwritten roles and rules. Roles involve position (Who is the breadwinner? Who takes out the garbage?). Roles always change as the patient needs to do less and shifts tasks to others. Rules are values; they can be about communication (Who can say what to whom?), emotion (Who is allowed to be sad?), education, sex, religion, and parenting.

Most important for people with hepatitis C are the family rules and values about health and illness. Problems arise when your family rules (or the rules of the family you grew up in) clash. Can you take time off if you have a cold or only if you're deathly ill? How do you handle the medical system?

> *My husband and I are having a hard time about my hepatitis C. He's an exercise nut and overdoses on vitamins. I do what my doctor tells me, and that's enough. My husband is constantly after me to change my lifestyle, and I get exasperated. I want to shout at him, "Leave me alone. I'll do it my way!"*
>
> *Janice*

Boundaries. Families create different boundaries. Some are so enmeshed that it's hard to tell where one member begins and another ends. They know how to pull together but need to learn how to allow outsiders to help. At the other end of the spectrum is the disengaged family where members have a high degree of autonomy and very little strong communication with each other. They need to learn how to draw closer, so they can hear each other and support one another. Most families, of course, fall somewhere in between these two extremes.

> *My sister would say, "Come on, let's go shopping." I didn't want to go because the interferon treatment made me tired. I knew she'd get mad if I had to leave in a couple of hours. So I'd say no. Then she'd glare at me and preach to me. She was always trying to control me.*
>
> *We had a blowout. We had been inseparable, and suddenly we weren't speaking.*
>
> Sally

Chronic illness can cause disorganization, but this crisis can open more options and choices as the family modifies and changes its rules and values.

> *My mom always said it was hard to believe someone was sick unless you could see a bleeding wound. But she stuck up for me all through my interferon treatment. Even though she's 85, and you'd think it would be hard for her to change, she was—and still is—the one person who understands what I'm going through.*
>
> Pete

Families also go through life stages that have their own issues of separateness and connectedness, from the birth of a child to taking care of elderly parents. When illness occurs, it can disrupt the normal tasks of these life stages. Suppose, for example, that hepatitis C strikes a parent of a teenager. The teenager will feel pulled by conflicting forces: the need to separate and develop a life with peers versus the need to pull closer to the family. In this setting the adolescent must cope with developing separateness and freedom and providing more help with household or other chores.

Communication and openness are the keys to improving the level of understanding within your family. When family members talk about a problem in terms of shifts in roles, rules and life stages, it diffuses the personal element. Usually, people feel hurt when a conflict arises because they think the other family members don't care about them. When you define the problem as a conflict in family roles, values, or degree of separation/connection, you can work toward a resolution.

Suppose, for example, that George wants his wife, Susan, to come with him to all his medical appointments. Meanwhile, Susan has had to take a part-time job to help pay the bills. Even though it's no one's fault, she's angry. Susan can't do it all, and her former role as the family's primary emotional support needs to be modified. Instead of blaming each other and feeling unloved, Susan and George talk about the role changes and come up with a compromise. Susan will go to the important medical appointments, and George will ask his sister to accompany him to the routine ones.

Do people want to change a family system? No, but illness brings unavoidable changes and, therefore, a feeling of loss of control. You can choose to be angry, or you can decide what can be changed and what cannot. How can we figure out a new system that's fair to everybody? What roles and values can we let go or modify?

Tools for Wellness: Some Practical Suggestions

Life-challenging illnesses, like hepatitis C, present opportunities for rethinking priorities. We may not always be able to cure the disease, but we can improve the quality of our lives. We can nourish ourselves by getting good medical and psychological care, exercising, eating nutritional foods, trying to live meaningful and useful lives, deepening relationships, having fun, and exploring our creative and spiritual sides.

Adapt an open and curious attitude when exploring these areas, and don't try all of them at once. Make changes gradually. Here are some suggestions from Pate-Willig and others:

CAUTION: Specific recommendations regarding diet, nutrition, and exercise may vary and should be evaluated and discussed with your physician.

Medical and Psychological Help. Put together your medical team with care. The treatment of hepatitis C is evolving and requires knowledge of specialized tests and treatments. Many doctors don't have much experience with hepatitis C, so find a gastroenterologist or hepatologist who does. Most medical centers have doctors who specialize in liver disease (hepatologists) or can recommend appropriate community specialists.

Although credentials are important, effective therapy may also be dependent upon the doctor-patient relationship. Make sure that the two of you are a good fit. This is a very individual matter. Do you like your doctor to tell you exactly what to do, or do you prefer to have more input with decision-making? Does the doctor answer your questions fully, or seem anxious to exit? Do the nurses and receptionist seem friendly and supportive?

If you need to see a mental health professional (psychologist, psychiatrist, social worker, professional counselor), get names from friends you trust and interview a few practitioners. Ask about their backgrounds and qualifications. Make sure they have experience in dealing with issues of chronic illness. They should be graduates of an accredited master's or Ph.D. program and licensed by the state as an independent practitioner or supervised by someone who is licensed.

Keep abreast of developments in hepatitis C research. The more you know, the better your decisions will be. (See the Resources section at the back of this book.) And finally, look at your own beliefs and attitudes about illness. Otherwise, you can't decide what works for you and what doesn't. We don't choose to be sick, but we can choose how we try to handle the situation.

Resources:

Bridges, William. *Transitions.* Reading: Addison-Wesley, 1980.

Clarke, Peter & Susan H. Evans. *Surviving Modern Medicine, How to Get the Best from Doctors, Family & Friends.* New Brunswick: Rutgers University Press, 1998.

Flach, Frederic, M.D. *Resilience: The Power to Bounce Back When the Going Gets Tough.* New York: Hatherleigh Press, 1997.

Kushner, Harold S. *When Bad Things Happen to Good People.* New York: Avon, 1981.

Travis, John W., M.D. and Regina Sara Ryan. *Wellness Workbook.* Berkeley: Ten Speed Press, 1988.

Many studies prove the importance of support systems. The results of one well-known study, reported in 1989 by psychiatrist David Spiegel and colleagues, showed that women with metastatic breast cancer who attended weekly group therapy sessions lived significantly longer than those who did not.[1]

Most of us benefit from a network of informal supportive relationships. Effective support always includes a sharing of emotions and feelings—a quality of reciprocity. Each person feels heard, validated, and has a sense of being able to draw upon that support, if necessary.

Formal support groups are useful because they provide a common experience for hepatitis C patients, information-sharing, a sense of not being alone, and a safe place to share feelings.

Resources: The Resources section at the back of this book lists national organizations that can direct you to local support groups in your area, phone networks, and online support groups. Also, your local hospital might be able to refer you to a group.

Hepatitis Magazine contains an updated directory of resources and organizations. Contact the magazine at 523 N. Sam Houston Pkwy. East, Suite 300, Houston, TX 77060, 281-272-2744; Email: editor@hepatitismag.com; Website: www.hepatitismag.com.

The Hepatitis Neighborhood offers a Support Group Search of almost 500 groups listed by state and a weekly Town Hall chat room (on specific topics) supervised by nurses. Website: www.hepatitisneighborhood.com.

Exercise and Nutrition. Physical movement not only strengthens your body, it helps your emotional state. If you can afford it, a personal trainer with experience in chronic illness is helpful. Hospitals often have cardiac or stroke rehabilitation experts who may be able to refer you to the right professional, but you don't need money to exercise. You can walk with a friend, rent yoga or Tai Chi videos, or try water exercise to avoid stress on painful joints. Be creative.

For information on nutrition, see Chapter 5, Taking Care of Yourself Nutritionally.

CAUTION: Consult your doctor before you begin any exercise program or make dietary changes.

Feeling Useful/Having Fun. We need a sense of meaning and purpose in our lives. We also need to have fun and play. Look for activities that create joy, hope, and a sense of living fully.

I'd always been a workaholic, but I started to question that kind of life when I learned I had hepatitis C. I didn't even like my job!

I started to try some new things like meditation. Then I got into art therapy and got really excited. One day I made a sand tray containing images of my life. In it, I put a house without a roof because my nice sub-

urban dream had blown up. I made a monster in a cage, because I felt like a monster, and a treehouse with the goddess Diana, who was the powerful part of me. I made a bridge that meant I was trying to get somewhere—paradise, a stream, lots of unconscious images.

I changed jobs. I played more. I ate healthier foods. As I look back now, I see that I'm in paradise. I crossed the bridge!

Maria

Ask yourself these questions: What is important to me? How am I acting on the important things in my life? How can I continue to have a meaningful existence within the limits of my health and energy levels?

Resources:

Anderson, Greg. *50 Essential Things to Do When the Doctor Says It's Cancer.* New York: Penguin, 1993.

LeShan, Lawrence. *Cancer As a Turning Point.* New York: Penguin, 1994.

Topf, Linda Noble with Hal Z. Bennett. *You Are Not Your Illness.* New York: Fireside, 1995.

Playing helps you recapture joy. "Like humor, a good joyful experience does as much for your sense of well-being as a good physical workout," says Pate-Willig. It requires flexibility and a commitment to explore options. If you can't climb mountains anymore, investigate handicapped-accessible trails or rent travel videos. Open yourself to new experiences. If you've never explored poetry, for example, now may be the time to visit your neighborhood library.

"Learn to live mindfully," says Pate-Willig. "Ask yourself: 'Do I notice the people chattering at my dinner table, and am I grateful for my family? Do I savor the vivid colors of the vegetables I'm cutting? Do I stop for a moment during the day to notice that I feel good?'"

Exploring Your Creative and Spiritual Sides. Using the mind's capacity for healing includes visualization, relaxation, guided imagery, meditation, journal writing, and creative arts. All of these are ways to help the mind create a quieter atmosphere and to improve your quality of life.

Visualization, meditation, and relaxation create a sense of relaxed alertness and counteract the stress of daily living. Visit a bookstore and look over the tapes and videos. There are more than 30 methods, so the important thing is to find what makes you feel comfortable.

Resources:

Benson, Herbert and Miriam Klipper. *The Relaxation Response.* New York: Avon, 1976.

Kabat-Zinn, Jon. *Full Catastrophe Living.* New York: Dell, 1990.

Journal writing lowers stress levels and can be your best friend in the middle of the night when there's no one else to talk to. Write quickly, don't censor yourself, and find a safe place to keep your journal.

Resources:

Capacchione, Lucia. *The Well-Being Journal.* North Hollywood: Newcastle, 1989.

Remen, Rachel Naomi, M.D. *Kitchen Table Wisdom, Stories That Heal.* New York: Riverhead Books, 1996.

Creative art forms (painting, drawing, music, dance, poetry) are healing because you work with symbols and images to express feelings.

Resource: Capacchione, Lucia. *The Creative Journal.* North Hollywood: Newcastle, 1989.

At first, after the diagnosis, I went a little crazy with therapies. I mean, I did it all—talk therapy, yoga, you name it and I did it. I ran myself ragged keeping up with all the appointments.

Finally, I decided it was too messy. I wanted to play. I took a dance weekend, and there it was. When I danced, I got to the stillness inside me. For me, dance relates to life and the creative process. Staccato movements, for example, meant I was having trouble with boundaries, with saying no. It became a metaphor for all of my life, and I began to feel healing on all levels.

Then we moved, and when I was going through boxes, guess what I found? A pair of little ballet slippers! I had completely forgotten that as a kid I had taken dance lessons—and loved them.

Sara

Guided imagery is a specific kind of relaxation and movement using the mind's own images. Most mental health professionals who deal with illness can assist you in creating an individual tape that works for you. A prerequisite is to practice relaxation so you can access guided imagery. The technique uses all five senses and works best when it's tailored to you. Not everyone sees images, for example. If that's the case with you, the therapist will use sounds or smells instead.

My ALT counts were high—in the 500s, so I went on interferon. It sounds a little far out, but I started to do this white light meditation. I visualized the interferon working on the hepatitis. Then my viral counts lowered to zero.

I visualized the interferon, like white knights assisting my immune system. B.I.S., Bill's Immune System. I saw a whole army of three million knights in shining armor!

Bill

Even if you don't hold formal religious beliefs, you can tap into your spirituality, says Pate-Willig. "Think back to your feelings at the birth of your child, or when you suddenly came upon a bed of glorious wildflowers. Spirituality connects you with a sense of something larger than the self."

If I had had to face death the year I was diagnosed, I would have felt I never lived. I was terrified, and I would have been angry with lots of regrets.

But as I got sicker, I had to go on disability. That gave me the time to explore, and I found out I could meditate, become still, and have a connection to a higher power. Now that I've had a chance to live fully, somehow I'm not as frightened of death.

Steve

Illness, however, can also present a theological challenge. According to Dr. House, some patients "go through a crisis of faith. People who've gone to church all their lives may suddenly feel rejected, alone and abandoned, angry with God, or feel this illness is punishment for some unknown sin. Their social network is centered on their church, so if they lose this, they lose a lot. I recommend that they talk to their clergy or to the hospital chaplain."

"Spiritual distress," says Rev. Julie Swaney, Chaplain at the University of Colorado Health Sciences Center, "occurs when a person's faith or spirit is suddenly full of holes. Everything you believe in is gone. You've lost your value system, and you feel alone. But one of the gifts of illness is the way it opens us up to life. People reassess relationships, values, their sense of time, of what's important. Spirituality has to do with how we make meaning out of our experiences. Embrace what works for you."

Resources:

Benson, Herbert, M.D., with Marg Stark. *Timeless Healing, The Power and Biology of Belief.* New York: Scribner, 1996.

Byock, Ira, M.D. *Dying Well, Peace and Possibilities at the End of Life.* New York: Riverhead Books, 1997.

Frankl, Victor E. *Man's Search for Meaning.* New York: Simon & Schuster, 1984.

Kushner, Harold S. *When All You've Ever Wanted Isn't Enough.* New York: Simon & Schuster, 1986.

Finally, one last word on being good to yourself: Take small steps to wellness slowly, over time. There is no correct formula. You may move back and forth, concentrating first on one area, then another—whatever works!

There is no grief which time does not lessen and soften.

Cicero

Reference

1. David Spiegel, M.D. *Living Beyond Limits.* (New York: Random House, 1993), p. 79.

7

TAKING CARE OF
YOURSELF FINANCIALLY
An Overview

Hey, this hepatitis C thing is tough. I get so tired, I almost fall asleep driving my truck. I've learned to pull over and take a quick nap. Just a few minutes, then I'm okay again.

I told my bosses I had hepatitis C. They nodded and said all the right things, but hey, it doesn't matter. I still have to do my job or I'm out. And if I'm out, I don't have health insurance. Then I can't afford interferon. But if I'm on interferon, I'm tired and I'm having trouble doing the work.

It's a Catch-22 situation, all right.

Tim

LIKE TIM, you may feel too sick to work, but you can't quit because you need to hold on to your health insurance. Or you're getting so many medical bills, you're worried about paying the mortgage. Any chronic illness can put a dent in your budget.

Each one of you, however, faces a different situation. This chapter presents a general overview of financial issues and supplies you with resources to help you find your own solutions.*

We'll cover:

- Cost of Treatment
  Ongoing Medical Care
  Antiviral Treatment
  Transplantation Costs
- Private Health Insurance
  Selecting Health Insurance
  Types of Private Health Insurance: Managed Care or Fee-for-Service
  HMOs
  PPOs
  Fee-for-Service Plans
- Government Health Insurance
  Medicare
  Medicaid
  Veterans Administration (VA)
- When You're Too Sick to Work: Applying for Disability
  Short-Term Disability Leave
- Disability Insurance
  Social Security Disability Insurance (SSDI)
  Supplemental Security Income (SSI)

*Note: This chapter is an overview, not an exhaustive treatment of financial options and programs. It does not provide legal advice; always contact agencies and companies for specific information and consult a lawyer for legal advice in specific cases.

Cost of Treatment

Ongoing Medical Care Costs. If you have a chronic illness, like hepatitis C, you have to consider the cost of lifelong medical care. At the very least, you need regular exams and blood tests to monitor your liver functions. For stable patients, the minimum recommendation is an annual physical examination and blood tests twice a year. You may also need a liver biopsy every three to five years. Ask your doctor what he or she recommends.

*In the past year I've had a liver biopsy and a blood clotting problem
that landed me in the emergency room and intensive care unit overnight.
That cost big time.*

*I've got health insurance, so I didn't worry until I heard at my hep-
atitis C support group that some insurance companies put a $1 million
lifetime cap on their policies. It seemed like a fortune until I started to
add up just this year's medical expenses. I finally called my company and
found out my cap is $2 million. What a relief!*

Susie

Antiviral Treatment Costs. Interferon treatment is costly. For
information, you may contact Schering-Plough Corporation, the manufacturer of INTRON® A (interferon alfa-2b, recombinant), PEG-
INTRON™ (peginterferon alfa-2b), and REBETRON™ combination
therapy; Hoffmann–La Roche, Inc., the manufacturer of ROFERON®-
A (interferon alfa-2a, recombinant) and PEGASYS® (peginterferon alfa-
2a); or Amgen, the initial manufacturer of INFERGEN® (interferon-
alfacon-1). (At the time of this writing, InterMune Pharmaceuticals,
Inc. was in the process of acquiring Infergen.) Phone numbers and
websites are listed in the Resource section below.

If you need help to pay for treatment, you, your doctor, or a family
member may contact the pharmaceutical company's reimbursement
search and financial assistance program to see if you qualify for aid.

Resource: For information about Schering-Plough's medications,
call 1-800-222-7579; website: www.schering-plough.com.

Schering's Commitment to Care℠ Program, 1-800-521-7157, offers
help in finding coverage, cost-sharing, and the providing of drugs to
indigent people. Have this information ready when you call:

1. name and address of your prescribing physician
2. diagnosis, prescribed drug therapy, and schedule
3. financial information: recent 1040 form, pay stub, Social Security
   number

Resource: For information about Roche's medications, call cus-
tomer service at 1-800-526-0625; website: www.rocheusa.com.

If you need help to pay for treatment, your doctor may contact Roche's ONCOLINE Reimbursement Assistance Program at 1-800-443-6676.

Resource: For information about INFERGEN®, contact Inter-Mune; website: www.intermune.com.

You might also consider enrolling in a study. Pharmaceutical companies often sponsor studies of promising new treatments; in many cases, the sponsor covers all costs of treatment. Be sure you understand exactly what the study involves, before you sign up for it. Ask your doctor for information or call a major research center or medical school near you (see Chapter 14, Research Trends).

Transplantation Costs. The hospital's financial coordinator will be on your transplant team to help you figure out how you can afford the procedure. There are many costs involved: tests and consultations before the operation, the transplant operation itself, hospitalization, and follow-up care and medications.

According to Fabi Imo, Coordinator, Transplant Financial Services at the University of Colorado Health Sciences Center, the charges for liver transplantation (from admission to discharge, but not including before or after care) vary widely, from $50,000 to more than $1 million. The average charge is approximately $200,000. Costs vary widely around the country.

"Transplantation and living donor liver transplantation are more accepted medical procedures now so they are covered by more insurance companies," says Imo. "Presently, Medicare and our state of Colorado Medicaid approve living donor transplantation because it is no longer considered an experimental procedure.

"Work with your hospital transplant financial coordinator to explore all your options. People often have insurance benefits they're not aware of. For example, some patients are covered for travel, lodging, and mileage costs."

According to Imo, sometimes patients who need financial help find themselves in a "Catch-22" situation. If you are disabled by liver disease and apply for Social Security Disability Insurance, a federal program, it takes 24 months (starting from the date you became eligible) for Medicare to become effective. Medicare does pay for liver transplants, but you may not be in a condition to wait two years.

"Another 'Catch-22' situation is the biggest problem I see," says Imo. "If the patient is over the minimum eligibility level, he or she will not qualify for Medicaid. And even if you have Medicaid, not all state Medicaid programs will cover a liver transplant."

Not all private insurance policies cover transplants, and both private and government health insurance impose certain criteria. For example, people who have additional medical problems, such as a heart condition, a malignancy, or HIV, may find themselves excluded from coverage.

In addition to determining insurance coverage for the transplant procedure itself, it's also important to look at your prescription drug benefit and how it covers immunosuppressive drugs. According to Imo, "The medications probably are the largest financial expense out of the patient's pocket. Post-transplant immunosuppressive medicines can be thousands of dollars a month." If you need help with medication costs, talk to your transplant coordinator about possible resources, such as pharmaceutical companies and other organizations.

Note: Medicare recently eliminated its former three-year time limit for coverage of post-transplant immunosuppressive medicines and now pays 80 percent of immunosuppressive drug costs for the lifetime of the transplanted organ. This policy applies to all Medicare-entitled beneficiaries who meet all of the other program requirements for coverage under this benefit.

Adding to direct costs are many indirect expenses. Patients sometimes forget to allow for organ recovery costs or travel and lodging for family members, childcare, and so on. It's important to plan ahead.

Finally, cautions Imo, it's important for patients to be involved with insurance companies. Know the name and phone number of your case manager, and always inform your financial coordinator and your liver transplant team immediately if you change insurance companies.

Resource: A 48-page booklet by the United Network for Organ Sharing (UNOS) discusses a number of topics, including financing transplantation. For a copy of *What Every Patient Needs to Know,* call 1-888-TXINFO1 (1-888-894-6361). The book also appears on the UNOS website: www.unos.org.

Resource: Another booklet, written by volunteers and distributed by the Organ Donor Program, may be helpful. For your free copy of *Finger in the Dike, Or: How to Raise $140,000 for Organ Transplant Surgery in Less Than Four Weeks,* call 1-800-452-1369 and ask for the Organ Donor Program.

Resource: The American Liver Foundation (ALF) has established a Liver Transplant Fund that provides professional administration, at no cost, for funds raised on behalf of patients to help pay for medical care and associated transplantation expenses. For information, call 1-800-GO-LIVER or 1-888-4-HEP-ABC.

Private Health Insurance

Selecting Private Health Insurance. When you have a chronic illness like hepatitis C, you must select your health insurance carefully:

- Read your policy before signing it. Ask questions. If there is any part you don't understand, get help.
- Make sure your plan allows you to see doctors who are experts in hepatitis C: gastroenterologists, hepatologists, and transplant physicians.
- Understand the restrictions and make sure they won't affect the quality of your care. For example, does the policy cover emergency rooms, experimental treatments, drugs like interferon? What happens if you're out of town and you need medical help?
- Is there a lifetime limit or cap on treatment or drugs? A million dollars may sound high, but is it too low for a chronic condition?
- Use common sense in assessing a medical policy. When you have hepatitis C, you have to plan ahead for extra medical care, even though you may never need it.
- Check to see if your policy pays based on "reasonable and customary" fee schedules. Policies that use fee schedules may not pay the entire bill if they feel that your doctor or hospital does not charge "reasonable" rates.
- Know any managed care provisions in your policy. Do you have any particular doctor or hospital that you are required to use? If you use a "preferred provider," will the insurance cover a larger share?

Types of Private Health Insurance: Managed Care or Fee-for-Service. Private health insurance policies fall into two categories: (1) managed care, or (2) fee for service. Managed care plans limit your choice of physician, but usually cost less. Managed care options include Health Maintenance Organizations (HMO) and Preferred Provider Organizations (PPO).

Fee-for-service policies usually provide the freedom to choose your doctor, but they often are more expensive. Look at the following factors when comparing cost of fee-for-service policies:

- monthly premiums—what the insurance costs each month
- annual deductible—how much you have to pay out of your pocket each year before the policy will pay benefits
- coinsurance—what percentage you have to pay that your insurance will not cover, usually 20 to 30 percent
- out-of-pocket maximum—the amount that you pay in coinsurance before the insurance company will begin to pay at 100 percent
- policy maximum—the maximum amount that insurance will pay over the lifetime of the policy

Whether you choose a managed care or traditional fee-for-service plan, be sure you understand how your plan works and the appeal process. If you're dissatisfied with your insurance policy, you may always review these issues with your State Commissioner of Insurance.

HMOs. Under HMO plans you have a primary care physician, a gatekeeper, who coordinates your care and decides if you should be referred to a specialist. This plan is the least costly but the most limiting in terms of freedom of choice. Because the goal is to keep costs at a minimum, your access to specialists, tests, medications, or hospital care may be restricted. It's important to do a thorough check on limitations.

PPOs. You may choose a doctor within the provider network and get 90 to 100 percent coverage of your costs or choose a doctor outside the network and receive a smaller percentage of the cost, usually 70 percent.

Fee-for-Service Plans. Usually, the choice of doctor is totally yours, but these plans are typically the most expensive. Patients with chronic hepatitis C who are exploring fee-for-service plans should choose a major medical policy that offers subspecialty physician services and adequate hospital coverage.

The insurance company usually pays 80 percent of the bill, and you pay 20 percent up to a total amount designated by your policy. Hospital and physician fees that the insurance company deems unreasonable may not be fully reimbursed.

Resource: To help consumers with the process of choosing a suitable health-care plan, check out two government websites: the Quality Inter-agency Coordination Task Force at www.consumer.gov/quality-health/index.html and the Department of Health and Human Services at www.healthfinder.gov/smartchoices/qualitycare/default.htm.

Resource: For help in evaluating health insurance plans, call the National Committee for Quality Assurance at 1-800-839-6487 for a personalized list of accredited HMOs in your area or visit website to view *Choosing Quality: Finding the Health Plan That's Right for You* (archives section): www.ncqa.org.

Resource: Another useful booklet is *Checkup on Health Insurance Choices,* AHCPR #93-0018, by the Agency for Health Care Policy and Research: 1-800-358-9295.

Resource: In 1996, Congress passed the Health Insurance Portability and Accountability Act (Public Law #104-191), sponsored by Senators Edward Kennedy and Nancy Kassebaum. This act includes many significant health insurance reforms.

Some highlights of the act include: (1) "portability" provisions, (2) increased availability of coverage, and (3) expansion of COBRA continuation coverage benefits. The "portability" provisions are designed to eliminate the fear that employees will lose their health insurance if they change jobs.

You may request a copy of the act and its accompanying conference committee report from your U.S. representative or senator. Also, as with other legislation of this type, government agencies, such as the Labor Department, the Internal Revenue Service, and the Department of Health and Human Services, will issue regulations to implement the act's provisions. In addition, almost all states will have to make changes in state legislation to comply with the act. For information, call your state legislators and your state insurance department.

Resource: Some states have set up risk-sharing pools to enable people who are otherwise uninsurable to purchase health insurance. Colorado, for example, has the Colorado Uninsurable Health Insurance Plan (CUHIP). State insurance laws differ, so call your state insurance department for specific information. If you have difficulty locating your state insurance department, contact the National Association of Insurance Commissioners for the listing: 816-842-3600. Website: www.naic.org

Government Health Insurance

CAUTION: Laws and regulations change over time. Double-check your facts with the agency involved. Only the agency itself can give you up-to-date, accurate material.

There are some situations when Medicare may eventually end, based on Social Security Disability Insurance (SSDI) eligibility. Also, the effects of work on benefits [SSDI and Supplemental Security Income

(SSI)] and Medicare/Medicaid are complicated and different depending on what benefit you get. The best thing to do is to call the Social Security Administration before you or your spouse works to see what the specific effects will be on your cash benefits and/or medical coverage.

This chapter does not give legal advice and is not a substitute for the professional services of an attorney. Always consult a lawyer when legal issues are involved.

Medicare. At age 65, you may be eligible for medical insurance for hospital and other medical services. If you receive Social Security disability benefits for 24 consecutive months (see following section), you also may qualify for Medicare.

Medicare has two parts. Hospital insurance (Part A) covers inpatient hospital care. You already paid for this as part of your Social Security and Medicare taxes when you were working. Medical insurance (Part B) pays for doctors' services, prescriptions, and some outpatient facility and doctor visits. Part B is optional, and you'll be billed monthly for your premium.

If you are not already getting Social Security benefits, sign up for Medicare at your local Social Security office three months before you become 65, and you'll receive your Medicare card. Ask about enrollment periods. If you are getting Social Security benefits, you will automatically be enrolled, and you will receive your card in the mail. You may also want to purchase a Medigap policy, or HMO, or other Medicare supplement (private insurance that fills in some of the "gaps" in Medicare's coverage).

Resources: Call the Centers for Medicare and Medicaid Services (CMS) Medicare Hotline (1-800-638-6833) or access its website (www.medicare.gov) to order publications, such as the *Medicare & You* handbook, and to get more information on Medigap supplemental insurance.

If you have a low income and few resources, you may qualify for state aid to help pay for Medicare premiums and some other expenses; ask for CMS's *Guide to Health Insurance.* You may also call the Department of Social Services.

Medicaid. Medicaid is a federal-state health program for people with low assets and incomes. At present, state social services departments administer the program. To apply, call your county social services department.

Veterans Administration (VA). For questions about medical benefits and disability, veterans may call the Veterans Administration Regional Office.

Resource: Dial this number and your call will be automatically directed to your regional office: 1-800-827-1000.

When You're Too Sick to Work: Applying for Disability

As hepatitis C progresses to the stage of cirrhosis, you may be less capable of functioning at home or on the job. In general, this occurs only in patients who have had the disease for many years and who have cirrhosis and signs of worsening liver function.

Our goal in this section is to provide you with a general overview of the available options for disability benefits and the process involved. For those who wish to consider applying for disability benefits, the process varies depending on your income, personal situation, and insurers or government programs.

CAUTION:

1. Laws and regulations change; unexpected circumstances arise. It's best to double-check your facts with the company, agency, or organization involved. Medical social workers can help direct you to the appropriate agencies or programs.
2. Keep a file with copies of all your medical records. Begin right now, if you haven't already done so. Always keep your EOBs (Explanation of Benefits) sent to you by your insurance company. The EOB is the document that explains what the medical provider and/or hospital is paid and contains a description of payment procedures.
3. Start a journal. Keep track of your symptoms and how they affect your daily tasks. This documentation will help you explain your symptoms to your doctor and will be important later if you ever have to file for disability.
4. This chapter does not give legal advice and is not a substitute for the professional services of an attorney. Consider consultation with a lawyer when legal issues or hearings are involved.

Resource: Call the American Bar Association at 312-988-5000 for your state's lawyer referral service number or check your phone book. Attorneys specialize in different areas, such as disability or insurance, so explain your specific problem. If you can't afford a lawyer, contact your local Legal Aid Society or a law school that sponsors a student association offering free legal advice. Your local United Way may also direct you to possible sources of legal help.

Short-Term Disability Leave. Become familiar with your company's policies. Some companies offer paid short-term disability leave or allow you to use accumulated sick days. Companies usually require that a doctor accurately assess the nature of your symptoms and verify that you are disabled. The diagnosis of hepatitis C or treatment with interferon and other antiviral medications are not sufficient, in and of themselves, to necessarily justify disability.

> *I was exhausted when I started taking interferon. My sister had died recently, and I thought it was depression that had me so tired. My doctor told me I had beginning cirrhosis, and I was so sick I needed to take some time off from work.*
>
> *I was incredulous. Taking time off was for operations! That was my own denial, my survival system. I was amazed that my company did approve leave—and I was paranoid. I expected surveillance cameras to sneak up on me. When I finally went back to work, it was part time, then full time. It was rough. I was achey; I had headaches. I just stayed in my cubicle and did what I had to do.*
>
> *I was afraid of losing my job. I didn't know my rights. I thought if I had six absences in a row, I'd be out the door.*
>
> *Joe*

If you are an eligible employee and you or your family member (child, parent, spouse) becomes seriously ill from advanced hepatitis C, the Family and Medical Leave Act allows you to take up to 12 weeks of unpaid leave each year. Workers returning from leave must be restored to their original jobs or equivalent jobs with the same pay, benefits, and working conditions.

Resource: For more information and to find out if you are an eligible employee under the act, call the nearest office of the Wage and Hour Division, listed in most telephone directories under U.S. Government, Department of Labor, Employment Standards Administration. Ask for copies of these publications: WH Publication #1420, *Your Rights Under the Family and Medical Leave Act*; WH Publication #1421, *Compliance Guide to the Family and Medical Leave Act*, U.S. Department of Labor,

Wage and Hour Division, Dec. 1996; and Fact Sheet No. ESA 93-24, U.S. Department of Labor Program Highlights, *The Family and Medical Leave Act of 1993.*

Resource: The 1990 Americans with Disabilities Act (ADA) prohibits job discrimination against "qualified individuals with disabilities." Employers covered under the act must make a "reasonable accommodation" for such persons depending on the particular facts in each case and on whether or not it imposes "due hardship" on the employer. "Reasonable accommodations" apply to the area of attendance and leave policies. To see if the ADA covers you and your employer and to get more specific information on the provisions of the act, call the President's Committee on Employment of People with Disabilities Job Accommodation Network at 1-800-ADA-WORK or 1-800-526-7234.; email: jan@jan.icdi.wvu.edu; website: www.jan.wvu.edu.

Disability Insurance

If you're self-employed, you may have paid for your own individual disability insurance. If you work for a company, find out if you are eligible to enroll in your company's group disability coverage. Read the terms of coverage carefully.

> *When I went on disability, I was at my highest earning capacity. It's a good thing I couldn't take a less stressful job at my company for less money. I would have had to quit anyway, and then I would have shot myself in the foot because my disability was computed as a percentage of my paycheck. It's hard enough to live on what I did get—60 percent of what I was earning.*
>
> *Arthur*

Two Social Security Administration programs offer assistance if you have to file for disability: Social Security Disability Insurance (SSDI) and Supplemental Security Income (SSI).

CAUTION: Brief descriptions of the programs follow, but only the agency itself can give you up-to-date, accurate material. *Call the Social Security Administration and ask them to send you information about disability programs:* 1-800-772-1213. You can speak to a service representative between the hours of 7 a.m. and 7 p.m. on business days. Hearing-impaired callers using TTY equipment can call 1-800-325-0778 during the same hours.

Social Security Disability Insurance (SSDI). This insurance covers workers (and their children or surviving spouses). In order to qualify for this disability coverage on your own record, you must have worked long enough and recently enough to have made sufficient contributions to your Social Security account. You may also qualify on the record of a parent or as a disabled widow(er). Adults must have a physical and/or mental problem that prevents them from working for at least a year or that is expected to result in death. Benefits continue until a person is able to work and earn a certain amount of money again on a regular basis.

You may file a claim by phone, mail, or by visiting the nearest Social Security office. The claims process can take about 180 days while the agency obtains medical information and decides if the disability affects your ability to work. You'll be asked to provide your Social Security number and proof of age and citizenship if born abroad; names, addresses, and phone numbers of doctors, hospitals, clinics, and institutions that treated you and dates of treatment; names of all medications you are taking; medical records from your doctors, therapists, hospitals, clinics, and caseworkers; laboratory and test results; a summary of where you worked in the past 15 years and the kind of work you did; a copy of your W-2 Form (Wage and Tax Statement), or if you are self-employed, your federal tax return for the past year; dates of prior marriages if your spouse is applying.

Social Security will request medical records from your physicians and hospitals to document your disability. However, your application will be processed faster if you provide this information for them up front when you apply.

> *After my biopsy I had to acknowledge how sick I was. I had cirrhosis. I was so fatigued that I had no life outside of work. For the time I had left, this was not the kind of life I wanted. So I became more assertive. Instead of waiting for my doctor to suggest disability, now I suggested it.*
>
> *As long as I was ambulatory, I thought I wasn't disabled. But when I put my symptoms on paper, I had to accept my feelings. I wrote about my inability to concentrate, my depression, the aches and pains, the constant headaches—and I presented the list to my doctor.*

He said I was disabled, outlined restrictions, gave me a prescription, and I took it to my employer. The disability plan at our company required me to sign up for Social Security Disability Insurance also.

At first, Social Security denied my claim. I went to a lawyer for help. I wish I had gone to him earlier. He told me it wasn't unusual to be denied at first. Hepatitis C symptoms of fatigue are vague, subjective. We appealed.

Social Security asked for an independent medical evaluation. I was prepared. I had kept a log of activities I could do and those I could not do. I went armed with my biopsy report. I finally saw myself as an educator of what hepatitis C was all about. I got disability.

Nadine

The Social Security Administration recommends that you don't wait to file your claim, even if you don't have all this information right away. (There is a waiting period before benefits begin, so the sooner you apply, the better.) If you need someone's help, a family member, caseworker, or other representative can contact the agency for you.

After your application is complete, the Social Security office will review it to see if you're eligible. Then they'll send your application to the Disability Determination Services (DDS) office in your state. (Consult SSA Publication No. 05-10029, which lists five questions that determine disability.)

If the claim is approved, you'll receive a notice showing the amount of your benefit and when payments start. The amount of your benefit is based on your lifetime average earnings covered by Social Security, but workers' compensation benefits can affect your disability check. Your case will be reviewed periodically to see if you remain disabled. After two years from the date of onset of disability, you will be eligible for Medicare benefits, regardless of your age. If your claim is denied, a notice will explain why, and you will have opportunities to contest the decision.

Resource: Call the Social Security Administration at 1-800-772-1213 (website: http://www.ssa.gov) for copies of SSA Publication No. 05-10057, *Social Security Disability Programs Can Help;* No. 05-10029, *Social Security Disability Benefits;* No. 05-10153, *What You Need to Know When You Get Disability Benefits;* No. 05-10041, *The Appeals Process;* No. 05-10075, *Your Right to Representation.*

Resource: Jehle, Faustin F. *The Complete & Easy Guide to Social Security, Healthcare Rights & Government Benefits.* Boca Raton: Emerson-Adams Press, 1998.

Resource: Mathews, Joseph L. with Dorothy Berman. *Social Security, Medicare, and Pensions.* Berkeley: Nolo.com. 1999.

Supplemental Security Income (SSI). SSI is a Social Security Administration program that makes disability payments to adults and children with little or no income or resources. To get SSI, you must be 65 or older, blind, or disabled. According to SSA Publication No. 05-11000, *Supplemental Security Income,* disabled means you have a physical or mental problem that keeps you from substantial work and is expected to last at least a year or to result in death.

The basic SSI payment is the same all over the country, but some states add money to your check. Any income you or your spouse has may affect the check amount. Call the Social Security Administration for information.

> When I applied for SSI, it was as if I was fighting against my whole value system. I had dreams that I was a gunrunner in South America. It felt as though I was doing something wrong or breaking the law.
>
> I was barely making it before hepatitis C, and now that I'm exhausted all the time, I can't make it at all. What else can I do?
>
> *Sam*

If you qualify for SSI, in most states you will be able to get other aid from your state or county, such as Medicaid (which helps pay doctor and hospital bills), food stamps, or other social services. Call your local social services department or public welfare office.

If you get Medicare and have low income and few resources, you may qualify for help with some Medicare premiums or co-pays under the Qualified Medicare Beneficiary (QMB) or Specified Low-Income Medicare Beneficiary (SLMB) programs. Only your state can decide if you qualify. Contact your county Social Services.

Whether your income meets SSI requirements depends on some very specific criteria defining what's included in income and what's included as assets outlined in SSA Publication No. 05-11000, *Supplemental Security Income.*

Sometimes people can get both Social Security and SSI benefits. The rules that determine if you're disabled are the same for Social Security and SSI (refer to the previous section, Social Security Disability Insurance). You must be unable to do any substantial kind of work to be considered disabled under both programs.

If you think you are eligible for SSI, the Social Security Administration recommends that you file a claim right away, even if you don't have all the information at hand. The information you need includes your Social Security card or a record of your Social Security number; your birth certificate or other proof of age; proof of citizenship; information about the home where you live (such as mortgage, lease, landlord's name); information about your income and the things you own (such as payroll slips, bank books, insurance policies, car registration, burial fund records, etc.), and names, addresses, and telephone numbers of doctors, hospitals, and clinics.

Resource: Call the Social Security Administration at 1–800–772–1213 (website: http://www.ssa.gov). Hearing-impaired callers using TTY equipment, call 1–800–325–0778. Explain why you're calling and ask for helpful information and pamphlets, including SSA Publication No. 05–10057, *Social Security Disability Programs Can Help;* No. 05–11000, *Supplemental Security Income;* No. 05–10101, *Food Stamp Facts;* No. 05–10100, *Food Stamps And Other Nutrition Programs;* No. 05–11011, *What You Need to Know When You Get SSI;* and No. 05–11069, *You May Be Able to Get SSI.*

Resource: Jehle, Faustin F. *The Complete & Easy Guide to Social Security, Healthcare Rights & Government Benefits.* Boca Raton: Emerson-Adams Press. 1998.

Riches serve a wise man but command a fool.

English proverb

8

EVOLUTION OF TREATMENT FOR HEPATITIS C

The Interferon Story and Ribavirin

When I was diagnosed with hepatitis C, I panicked—especially when the doctor described interferon treatment to me. I had just read this book about how toxic our environment is, so I decided to try an alternative route: macrobiotic diet, vitamin supplements, changing my dental fillings from mercury to gold—the whole nine yards.

My ALT and AST levels went down some; the PCR test went down some. I thought I had hit the cure. But the next time I got tested, the scores crept up again. It turns out that hepatitis C spikes—up and down, high and low. I was into a much healthier lifestyle—and that was good—but I still had the virus.

I finally started interferon. My test levels went down and have stayed down. As far as I'm concerned, it's the only antiviral game in town.

Ted

Making treatment decisions can be a stressful process. You and your doctor will work together to decide on a treatment plan. But it helps to know as much as you can about your options.

The following Chapter 9 discusses the latest multi-center clinical trials of the emerging standard-of-care, pegylated interferons. In this chapter I'll cover the following topics about interferon and ribavirin:

- Overview
- Interferon Monotherapy
    - What Is Interferon?
    - Who Should Take Interferon?
    - Interferon Treatment
    - Types of Interferon
    - Measuring Response
- Interferon in Combination with Ribavirin
    - What Is Ribavirin?
    - Who Should Take Combination Therapy?
    - Combination Treatment
    - Measuring Response
- The Patient's Experience
    - Injections
    - Interferon Side Effects
    - Ribavirin Side Effects
- Treatment Tips from Patients
    - Interferon Monotherapy
    - Combination Therapy
- After Treatment, What Next?
    - Nonresponders and Relapsers
    - Re-Treatment with Combination Therapy
    - If You Are a Responder
    - Continuing Care
    - Vaccinations

NOTE: For information on pegylated interferons, the emerging standard-of-care, see Chapter 9.

Overview

As a patient with chronic hepatitis C, you may experience fatigue, loss of energy, loss of concentrating ability, and a sense of inadequacy in performing your daily activities. These symptoms, feelings, and attitudes may make you emotional or susceptible to periods of depression.

I encourage you to continue to remain physically active, pursue your occupation, socialize, and maintain proper nutrition. I also recommend regular exercise and a well-balanced diet supplemented with one multivitamin per day. (See Chapters 5 and 6 for more detailed suggestions on how to take care of yourself nutritionally and emotionally.)

Remember: Alcohol and hepatitis C don't mix. Avoid excessive alcohol intake; the combination of alcohol and hepatitis C may accelerate your liver disease. I discourage the daily drinking of alcohol or taking large amounts at any time.

However, alcohol use is socially acceptable, so many patients ask me if they can take a drink once in a while. If you're not willing to abstain completely from alcohol, you should at least limit your alcohol intake to less than two ounces a week.

Patients also question me about alternative therapies. A number of herbal remedies, teas, potions, over-the-counter products, and even acupuncture claim to be effective in treating liver disease and viral hepatitis, but none have been adequately studied. The use of these treatments to eradicate hepatitis C is not encouraged because their effectiveness is doubtful and their safety, in general, is unknown. In one recently published report, a Chinese herbal remedy marketed as a sedative and analgesic, Jin Bu Huan, was associated with severe liver injury in seven patients. Be sure to check with your doctor before taking any over-the-counter products or other substances (see Chapter 5, section on Herbs Harmful to the Liver).

Interferon Monotherapy

What Is Interferon? Scientists identified interferon in 1957 by demonstrating that cells infected with a virus secreted a substance that had the ability to protect other uninfected cells from becoming infected. This substance, interferon, is a naturally occurring protein whose name is derived from its ability to interfere with viral replication.

Since these early studies, the interferon story has become increasingly complex. Three classes of interferons, alpha, beta, and gamma, are currently recognized. Gamma interferon is ineffective against hepatitis

C. Beta interferon is less effective than alpha interferon. Alpha interferons are the most effective interferons in treating patients with hepatitis C.

Who Should Take Interferon? The criteria for selecting patients for treatment were developed in the first two controlled studies of interferon in treating hepatitis C (US Multi-Center Trial and NIH Trial, November 1989). These criteria center on three main issues: how long you've had the disease (chronicity), confirmation of a diagnosis of hepatitis C, and absence of severe liver injury (compensated liver disease). The initial criteria used were the following:

- persistently elevated ALT for at least six months
- liver biopsy compatible with diagnosis of chronic hepatitis
- no other serious underlying medical condition
- no evidence of hepatic failure (ascites, variceal bleed, encephalopathy)
- bilirubin < 4 milligrams/deciliter
- albumin > 3 grams/deciliter
- prothrombin time < 3 seconds prolonged beyond control
- platelet count > 70,000/microliter
- white blood count > 3,000/microliter, polymorphonuclear leucocytes (PMN) > 1,500/ microliter
- hemoglobin > 11 grams/deciliter

(For a full explanation of technical terms listed above, see Chapter 2.)

Current criteria for treatment and standard-of-care also require that patients test positive for the hepatitis C virus by antibody and HCV-RNA assay. In addition, emerging data indicate that patients with normal ALT and others with advanced liver disease may benefit from treatment.

Interferon Treatment. Interferon alfa-2b (INTRON® A, Schering-Plough) was the first interferon approved by the Food and Drug Administration (FDA) in the United States for the treatment of chronic hepatitis C. Interferon alfa-2a (ROFERON®-A, Roche) and interferon alfacon-1 (INFERGEN®, Amgen) have also been approved. On January 19, 2001, the FDA approved the first pegylated interferon, Peginterferon alfa-2b (PEG-INTRON™, Schering-Plough). As of August 2001, Peginterferon alfa-2a (PEGASYS®, Roche) awaits FDA approval. (Table 8A lists interferons approved or under review by the FDA.)

Non-pegylated interferon therapy is prescribed as three million units for Intron A or ROFERON®-A, or nine micrograms for Infergen given three times a week (tiw), usually Monday, Wednesday, and Friday, for up to 12 months. Investigators have tried higher doses, daily dosing, and longer courses of interferon with some improvements in overall response rates.

Types of Interferon. Existing data suggest that the alpha interferons are similarly effective in terms of the overall response rates of hepatitis C. Side effects are similar, but their frequency of occurrence varies slightly among the different interferons.

Measuring Response. Two factors appear to consistently predict a complete or sustained response (Figure 8A):

• The patient has an HCV genotype other than type 1.
• Plasma levels of HCV are below two million copies per milliliter.

(Some studies, but not all, suggest that young age also helps predict a positive response to interferon.)

How do you know when interferon is working? We measure its effectiveness in three ways:

1. ALT levels become normal. Hepatitis C is a liver disease, and the ALT reflects ongoing injury to the liver. Normalization of ALT implies that liver injury has stopped or is diminished.

TABLE 8A. TYPES OF INTERFERON.
Listed in order of introduction to market.

Type	Trade Name	Pharmaceutical
Interferon alfa-2b	INTRON®A	Schering-Plough
Interferon alfa-2a	ROFERON®-A	Roche
Interferon alfacon-1	INFERGEN®	Amgen
Peginterferon alfa-2b	PEG-INTRON™	Schering-Plough
Peginterferon alfa-2a	PEGASYS®	Roche

2. The hepatitis C virus (HCV-RNA) disappears from the blood, as measured by PCR assays.
3. A post-interferon treatment biopsy shows an improvement in the condition of the liver.

Looking at experimental statistics gives us important information, but when you are the person who's taking interferon, you want to know how to measure success or failure. Physicians have a special vocabulary, mainly based on measuring HCV-RNA, to describe response (Figure 8B):

- **Complete responder:** The patient has no detectable HCV-RNA in his or her blood during the last two months of treatment.
- **Nonresponder:** These patients do not respond to current antiviral treatment. HCV-RNA remains positive throughout therapy.

FIGURE 8A.   SUSTAINED RESPONSE TO INTERFERON MONOTHERAPY (%RNA NEGATIVE, 6 MONTHS POST-TREATMENT) IS MORE COMMON WITH NON–1 HCV GENOTYPES, LOW LEVELS OF RNA, AND LONGER DURATION (48 WEEKS) OF TREATMENT.[1]

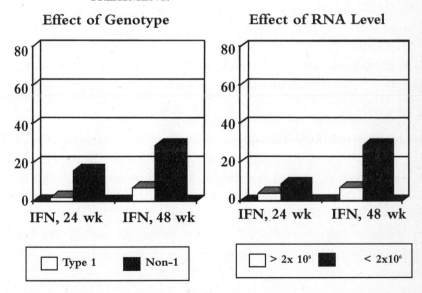

Measuring Response. Long duration (48 weeks) of treatment improves sustained response in type 1 and non–1 HCV genotypes.

FIGURE 8B. PATTERNS OF HCV–RNA RESPONSE

HCV-RNA x 10⁶ viral particles per ml

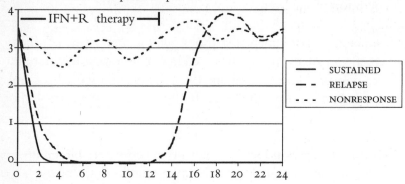

Legend 8B: The three main types of response of hepatitis C to antiviral therapy are shown. Sustained responders (solid black line), clear virus (HCV-RNA) from blood during therapy, usually within 3 months, and virus is undetectable throughout the remainder of treatment and post-treatment followup. Relapsers (dashed line) clear virus (HCV-RNA) from blood during therapy but HCV-RNA re-emerges once treatment has been stoppped. Nonresponders (dotted line) fail to clear virus both during and after treatment.

- **Relapse:** Complete responders, who are RNA negative at the end of treatment, are classified as relapsers when HCV-RNA becomes positive after treatment is stopped.
- **Sustained response:** Sustained responders are negative for HCV-RNA six months after treatment has been discontinued. More than 95 percent of sustained responders remain free of hepatitis C after years of follow-up and are likely "cured."
- **Improved liver histology:** In most studies, interferon therapy is associated with improvement in the condition of the liver cells. This improvement occurs not only in those who clear HCV-RNA but also in those who remain positive for the virus. Improved histology is due mostly to reduced inflammatory activity. Recent studies also suggest that interferon therapy may inhibit the production of substances that cause liver fibrosis.

Interferon in Combination with Ribavirin

In the first edition of this book (©1997) combination therapy with interferon plus ribavirin was under investigation and considered experimental. By the time of our second edition (©1999) the results of large multi-center, multinational trials indicated that the combination therapy of Intron® A and ribavirin was significantly better than monotherapy with Intron® A. Combination treatment, REBETRON™ (Schering-Plough), was approved by the Food and Drug Administration for relapsed patients in June 1998, for naïve patients (previously untreated with alpha interferon therapy) in December 1998, and it became the standard-of-care.

Currently, pegylated interferon plus ribavirin is emerging as the next standard-of-care. On July 26, 2001, the FDA approved the separate dispensing of ribavirin as REBETOL® (Schering-Plough) capsules, and on August 8, 2001, the FDA approved Peg-Intron for use in combination

FIGURE 8C. SUSTAINED RESPONSE TO INTERFERON + RIBAVIRIN (%RNA NEGATIVE, 6 MONTHS POST-TREATMENT) IS MORE COMMON WITH NON–I HCV GENOTYPES AND LOW LEVELS OF RNA.[1]

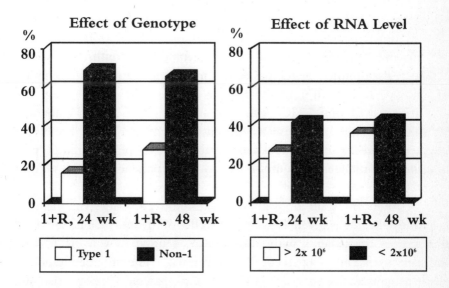

Measuring Response. Long duration (48 weeks) of treatment improves response in HCV genotype 1.

with Rebetol. As of August 2001, Pegasys (Roche) awaits FDA approval as monotherapy and in combination with ribavirin. (See Chapter 9 for more information on pegylated interferons).

What Is Ribavirin? Ribavirin is a nucleoside analogue of guanosine and has antiviral activity against a variety of DNA and RNA viruses. In addition, ribavirin modifies the immune response and enhances the antiviral activity of interferon. The exact mechanism of action of ribavirin against hepatitis C is unknown and under investigation. Ribavirin, when used as monotherapy, has no beneficial effect on serum HCV-RNA levels; it is effective only in combination with interferon.

Who Should Take Combination Therapy? Pegylated interferon will likely replace standard interferon as the companion drug with ribavirin in future treatment (see Chapter 9). Candidates for combination treatment are essentially those as described above for interferon monotherapy. Because ribavirin breaks down red blood cells, hemoglobin concentration should be greater than 12 gms/dl (grams per deciliter) in women and 13 gms/dl in men. Additionally, candidates should

- have platelet count > 100,000
- have no active cardiovascular disease
- practice adequate contraception to avoid pregnancy

Combination Treatment. Standard combination treatment (Rebetron) is Intron A 3MU tiw + ribavirin 1 to 1.2 g/day. As previously noted, pegylated interferon is likely to replace Intron A in future regimens. Optimum duration of treatment is six months for patients infected with non-1 genotypes and 12 months for patients infected with genotype 1. As with monotherapy, the likelihood of sustained response is greatest with non-1 HCV genotype and low RNA levels (Figure 8C).

The sustained response for patients with non-1 HCV genotypes given 24 weeks and 48 weeks of therapy were 69 percent and 66 percent. The sustained responses for genotype 1 patients were 16 percent and 28 percent.

Two recent trials of pegylated interferon plus ribavirin included groups of patients given 48 weeks of Rebetron treatment. The sustained responses for patients with non-1 HCV genotypes were 61 percent (Pegasys trial) and 79 percent (Peg-Intron trial). The sustained responses for patients with genotype 1 HCV were 37 percent (Pegasys trial) and 33 percent (Peg-Intron trial). Long-term follow-up indicates that more than 95 percent of sustained responders remain free of HCV, suggesting that these patients may be "cured."

The addition of ribavirin to interferon was a major step forward in the treatment of hepatitis C. Use of this combination was considered standard-of-care (year 2000-2001). The combination of pegylated interferon plus ribavirin is an extension of this therapy and is likely to be the new standard-of-care for years to come (see Chapter 9).

Measuring Response. The definitions of response (non-response, relapse, complete and sustained) are similar to those used above for interferon monotherapy.

The Patient's Experience

Many patients are nervous about interferon injections and concerned about dealing with side effects of treatment.

Injections. In my experience, patients quickly learn how to give themselves injections. Most people think of the deep muscle injections they get for flu shots, and they panic about doing this to themselves. Interferon injections are much easier to administer because they are subcutaneous. Subcutaneous means you have to get the needle only under the skin and not deep into muscle.

> *I was really nervous about learning how to give myself a shot. When I came into the office, the nurse was looking all around for an orange to practice on. She never did find it. So we used the pad on the exam table, then a tissue box. It was funny, and it made me laugh—something I never expected to happen.*
>
> *The first couple of times I did it myself at home, I put the needle in too horizontally. I was going push, push, push and nothing happened. I got awful bruises.*
>
> *Back to the nurse. She told me to pinch my skin between two fingers, hold the syringe like a dart and go in straight at a 90° angle. That worked!*
>
> *Marla*

It's important that you ask questions and practice injections under a nurse's supervision until you feel comfortable. You should be taught about storing and preparing the drug for injection, sterile technique, how to pick injection sites, and how to dispose of needles. Be sure to ask for the helpful teaching material and videotapes that pharmaceutical companies give to physicians for their patients' use.

I recommend that the first shot be given in the office. Although it's highly unlikely for a patient to have an immediate adverse reaction, we observe the patient for a couple of hours.

Interferon Side Effects. Each person reacts differently to interferon. The most common complaints are flu-like symptoms. Why? When you get an actual case of the flu, your body fights back by sending interferon to attack the invader. Interferon is at least partially responsible for the tired, achy, and feverish symptoms.

Some people don't have many symptoms during interferon treatment; other people get chills, muscle aches, nausea, even diarrhea. These symptoms usually subside after the first few weeks. Weight loss is also a common side effect, but it tends to persist throughout the course of therapy. Some patients are able to maintain their weight and improve their energy by using supplements, such as Ensure Plus®, Resource®, and Suplena®.

To help with side effects, I recommend two regular strength Tylenol® just before you take the injection. Side effects may also be reduced if you're well hydrated before and after the injection (two glasses before an injection and about two-and-a-half quarts of fluid a day).

For fatigue, it may help to have a daily nap or rest period. Paradoxically, some patients feel their fatigue is relieved by daily activity, including exercise. Eat small, more frequent meals if you're losing your appetite. To avoid skin reactions, rotate the injection sites.

During interferon therapy you will need frequent blood tests. The main reason for doing these blood tests is to be certain your blood counts are adequate. Interferon reduces the white blood cell count and the platelet count. This effect of interferon is directly related to the dose used; higher doses cause a greater lowering of the counts. Sometimes the dose of interferon may need to be reduced or even discontinued.

Particularly distressing side effects that occur in a minority of patients include depression, mental changes, and hair loss. Depression on interferon usually occurs in patients with a pre-treatment history of depression. However, it can occur in any patient, bears close supervision, and may require reducing the dosage or even stopping treatment. In some cases, in order to continue interferon, your physician may prescribe medication to control symptoms of depression (Zoloft®, Elavil®,

Effexor®, or Prozac®). If hair is lost during treatment, it usually grows back after treatment stops. Your physician will monitor you closely to watch out for other rare side effects, including thyroid disease or the development of other autoimmune disorders (see Chapter 4).

Be sure to tell your doctor if any of these symptoms appear:

• thoughts of suicide
• thoughts of homicide
• sustained fever (greater than 102° F) or other signs of infection
• generalized rash
• any symptoms that are interfering with your daily activity

Interferon may affect your ability to fight infection. Do not undergo procedures, such as excessive dental work, without checking with your doctor first; your physician may decide to prescribe an antibiotic to protect you.

Generally, most people adjust well. I tell patients to keep busy, exercise, drink lots of water, rest when they need to, socialize. Focus on positive things. Above all, don't let interferon isolate you.

Ribavirin Side Effects. Breakdown of red blood cells (hemolysis) is a common side effect of ribavirin, necessitating dose reductions in approximately 5 to 10 percent of patients. This adverse reaction occurs early in treatment and typically stabilizes after the first four weeks. Rarely does a patient withdraw completely from therapy due to this reaction.

Other side effects that occur more frequently with combination therapy than with interferon monotherapy include shortness of breath, throat irritation, itching, rash, nausea, difficulty sleeping, and loss of appetite. Twenty to 26 percent of patients will require dose reductions related to any of the above side effects.

Treatment Tips from Patients

Here are some tips from hepatitis C patients who've gone through treatment. Remember, what works for one person may not work for you. Once you become familiar with these drugs, you'll find your own comfort level.

INTERFERON MONOTHERAPY

For me, drinking lots of water helped. If I didn't stay hydrated, I felt worse.

When my husband started interferon, it changed our lives. We weren't prepared for it. Interferon can be hard on the spouse, too. To be supportive, I had to plan things at a slower rate.

My husband and I used to ski all day long—black and double-black runs. We used to take 10 to 15 mile hikes. During treatment, I would have to encourage him to take a half-hour walk on flat ground—just to get him off the couch and outside.

I dropped 20 pounds because I had no appetite—and I'm pretty thin as it is. My stomach was... I don't know, I just couldn't seem to eat. You really have to make sure you eat, even if you have to take several smaller meals throughout the day.

Now that I'm off interferon, I'm drinking two of those instant breakfast mixes each day, and I've gained back 12 pounds!

I'm on five million units, and I'm able to continue to ride my bike 200 miles a week. If I can't ride, the effects of the interferon seem stronger.

The people in my support group decided the two major things that helped were to get a lot of rest and to have a positive attitude. What's really interesting is that in spite of the side effects, no one was sorry they had tried interferon.

Here's a tip that works for me. Take your thumb and press hard for 10 seconds on the place where you're going to inject. It numbs the skin a little bit.

I'm a fair bit more irritable. So I apologize and say I'm not feeling well. It's me, not you. I do a fair amount of apologizing.

It's a peculiar kind of headache. I call it the interferon headache. Also, it seems as though I'm more forgetful. All my friends tell me they forget things, too, that I'm just getting older. But it seems different to me. Now I write everything—and I mean everything—down!

One night I took an early bath and really soaked. Then I did the shot. My skin was so soft, the needle went right in. Don't do the reverse, though. Don't take a hot bath after the shot.

In the morning and at night, I feel nauseous. If I eat, the nausea goes away. I have to concentrate on eating. And if I eat right before or after an injection, I don't have side effects.

My hairdresser told me my hair was thinning out, but not to worry because it was so thick in the first place. When I stopped interferon, it all came back.

For me, the fatigue is the tough part. I got over the slight fever and upset stomach in the first couple of days. But I do get tired, and I just have to rest more. About midway through the treatment, I had to go on an antidepressant, and that's helped me a lot.

I've had to learn to say no. It's amazing how you can simplify your work life if you have no choice. And I've learned not to schedule too many appointments in one day. If I'm running from one thing to another, I'm wiped out at the end of the day.

COMBINATION THERAPY

I had a breakthrough on interferon, so my doctor put me on ribavirin right away. It took me weeks to adjust to the shortness of breath. When I walk fast—and I'm used to walking fast—I start to feel faint, like I'm going to pass out. Stairs are even worse.

My lower red blood cell count means I get less oxygen. I've learned to move slower, not to rush from one thing to another. Also, if I feel faint, I slow down and take deep breaths to get more oxygen in my system. On the plus side, my counts are down again!

This ribavirin really kicks my butt! I couldn't keep up at work. Finally, I told everyone what's going on. They still resent having to pick up some of the slack, but they're much more understanding.

I started combination therapy two weeks ago. I expected chills or something, but I didn't feel anything—maybe a little ache in my back. I notice I get winded easier, but I just ride my bike slower.

I've felt worse taking antibiotics for a sinus infection. Drinking a lot of water seems to help.

I had a hard time getting used to the ribavirin. I started to get nervous, anxious. I was very ragged, emotionally. Also, I lost weight. If I had known I'd feel better after a couple of months, I could have taken it in stride. I thought it would go on forever.

I was brushing my teeth when I saw something black on my tongue. When I looked closer at the mirror, there were lots of black spots. "My gosh," I thought, "I've got the plague, the Black Death!"

Turned out the spots were prominent veins. My doctor reduced my ribavirin dose, and the spots went away. My cough got better, too. But I've also noticed more dry skin, dry eyes, itching. I just keep putting ointments on everything.

I was so discouraged when my doctor reduced my dose. I thought it was all over. Then I found out that a woman in my support group went down to only four pills a day—and she cleared the virus. It's six months now, and she's still clear! That made me feel better.

I lost a lot of weight at first because the ribavirin made me queasy. I don't know why, but I was taking the pills on an empty stomach. Now I take them after I eat, and I drink lots and lots of water. I don't feel nauseous anymore.

Where do these rashes come from, especially the dry spots on my elbows? I get purplish bumps, like goose bumps—and they itch. Sometimes bathing in water with sea salts helps.

After Treatment, What Next?

When you finish the course of treatment your doctor prescribes, your response is categorized as non-response, complete, relapse, or sustained (see definitions above). Nonresponders fail to clear HCV-RNA during treatment and relapsers become RNA positive after treatment has stopped. Sustained responders normalize ALT, clear HCV-RNA on treatment, and remain RNA-negative after treatment has stopped. What your doctor recommends next depends on your initial response to treatment.

Nonresponders and Relapsers. For nonresponders, the first question is whether you took the interferon as prescribed. Did you miss doses? If so, why? Were the side effects intolerable? Were you able to take the full dose or was the dosage reduced? If the dosage was reduced, why? The answers to these questions tell the physician how to proceed.

If you missed doses and never received a full course of treatment, the treating physician must determine the reasons. Some patients experience intolerable side effects, and they could not comply with treatment. If that was the case, then re-treating with the same regimen isn't a likely option unless other treatments can be used to minimize side effects. For example, if the dosage was reduced or stopped due to depression, it may be possible to re-treat with combination therapy (including pegylated interferon plus ribavirin) after treating the depression. If the dose was reduced because of severe lowering of white blood cells or red blood cells, you may be able to tolerate re-treatment with either interferon or combination therapy by also taking drugs to increase white cells (Neupogen®) or red cells (Epogen®).

Doctors must address these and other issues because current protocols involving re-treatment usually use higher doses and long duration of the combination of pegylated interferon plus ribavirin (see Chapter 9). Obviously, patients intolerant to interferon therapy are not likely to tolerate these re-treatment protocols.

Re-Treatment with Combination Therapy. There are several studies that examined the effectiveness of re-treatment using the standard combination of interferon plus ribavirin in people who did not respond to an initial course of interferon monotherapy. A recent analysis evaluated nine controlled and 62 uncontrolled studies in which nonresponders were re-treated with six months of combination therapy. This analysis indicated that only 13.2 percent of nonresponders cleared hepatitis C. However, the rates of sustained viral clearance varied considerably, from 0 percent to 40 percent. In another study, 30.6 percent of patients who received 24 to 48 weeks of re-treatment with combination therapy sustained viral clearance.

Our own experience in Colorado with re-treating patients who did not respond to monotherapy has been encouraging. We recruited 96 patients into a prospective study of 48 weeks of re-treatment with Rebe-tron (5 million units of interferon, injected three times a week plus 1 to 1.2 grams/day of ribavirin). The study involved 67 men and 29 women. They ranged in age from 30 to 64. Sixty-eight percent had HCV geno-type 1, one of the most difficult genotypes to treat. Sixteen percent of those enrolled in the study had already developed cirrhosis. Thirty per-cent of those enrolled in the study experienced sustained viral remission after six months of post-treatment follow-up.

The data from all of these re-treatment trials indicate that the stan-dard combination of interferon plus ribavirin is effective in re-treating patients who previously failed interferon monotherapy. In the future, patients are likely to be retreated with the combination of pegylated interferon plus ribavirin (see Chapter 9).

If You Are a Responder. A sustained response is the most desir-able outcome after antiviral treatment. Most patients with a sustained response have cleared the virus from their blood and have improvement in their liver biopsy (fewer inflammatory cells and less damage).

Long-term sustained responders (more than three years) may have halted the progression of their liver disease and may have actually cleared hepatitis C completely. However, there is always the risk, albeit small, that hepatitis C may only be dormant and reactivate, flaring at a later date. Patients should continue to undergo periodic biochemical tests and physical examinations.

Continuing Care. Patients with hepatitis C are at risk for progres-sive liver injury, cirrhosis, complications of end-stage disease, and may ultimately require liver transplantation for survival. Additionally, these patients are at risk for developing liver cancer (hepatoma). Thus, general medical advice includes ongoing physical examinations by a physician and biochemical tests of liver function. Cirrhotic patients with hepatitis C may need periodic measurement of alpha-fetoprotein and ultrasound examinations to detect early liver cancer (see Chapter 11). You should understand that the combination of alcohol and hepatitis C can cause early progression to cirrhosis and liver failure. Active alcoholism is a contraindication to liver transplantation.

Vaccinations. The 1997 National Institutes of Health (NIH) guidelines indicate that hepatitis C patients should get vaccinated for hepatitis A and B. If they're not currently immune, I agree with these recommendations, but you should check with your physician before getting vaccinated, especially if you are on interferon monotherapy or combination therapy.

> *A drug is a substance which when injected*
> *into a guinea pig produces a scientific paper.*

> *Anonymous*

Reference

1. Figures 8A and 8C were created using data from Table 4 in the following article:
McHutchison, J. G., S. C. Gordon, E. R. Schiff, M. L. Shiffman, W. M. Lee, V. K. Rustgi, Z. D. Goodman, M. H. Ling, S. Cort, J. K. Albrecht for the Hepatitis Interventional Therapy Group. "Interferon alfa-2b Alone or in Combination with Ribavirin as Initial Treatment for Chronic Hepatitis C." *New England Journal of Medicine.* 1998;339:1485-1492.

9

PEGYLATED INTERFERONS
The Emerging Standard-of-Care

My first liver biopsy in 1998 showed cirrhosis, but I had no symptoms. When I asked my gastroenterologist what my life expectancy would have been if I hadn't found out I had hepatitis C, he told me five years—if I was lucky. That brought me up short!

I tried interferon monotherapy. Slowly, my liver functions went down, but not to normal, and my viral count never went down.

I realized I had to do something or by 50 I'd be dead. The hepatologist said I could try the new combination therapy. My liver enzymes went down to normal, but my viral load did not—and I had terrible side effects.

"It's not working. Take a break," the hepatologist said. "I've got some clinical trials coming up with pegylated interferon." I'm never doing this again, I thought. But when they called me for the HALT C[1] study last year, I decided I needed to do something to stay alive.

I'm nine months into the study, and three months ago the virus was undetectable. Even if I don't hold the response, I'm glad I enrolled. I've had hepatitis C since 1980—21 years—and this is the first time my liver has gotten a rest!

Emma

WHAT ARE YOUR OPTIONS if you have not yet started interferon or if you did not clear hepatitis C after a previous course of treatment? What will be the next standard-of-care?

Clinical investigators have been conducting research on pegylated (long-acting) interferons in large multi-center studies for several years. Recent results of these studies are hopeful and encouraging.

In this chapter I'll explain basic facts about pegylated interferons and discuss the study data so that you can work with your doctor to develop the best treatment plan for you. Here are the topics I'll cover:

• What Is Pegylated Interferon?
• Advantages of Pegylated Interferon
• How Pegylated Interferon Works
• Clinical Trial Results
• Monotherapy Trials (How Good Are Pegylated Interferons without Ribavirin?)
• Combination Trials (How Good Are Pegylated Interferons Combined with Ribavirin?)
• The Patient's Experience: Treatment with Pegylated Interferon Plus Ribavirin
• Treatment Tips from Patients on Pegylated Interferon Plus Ribavirin
• Treatment of Nonresponders or Relapsers (What Are Your Chances of Responding to Pegylated Interferon Plus Ribavirin?)
   Projected Results with Re-Treatment: Can We Peer into the Future?
• Alternatives to Pegylated Interferons Plus Ribavirin

Note: Refer to Chapter 8 for basic information on interferon, ribavirin, definitions of treatment response, and other patient issues.

What Is Pegylated Interferon?

The "peg" of pegylation is an abbreviation for polyethylene glycol, a biologically inert compound. Researchers are using PEG, a substance that thickens lipstick and shampoo products, to improve the effectiveness of medicines. Your body basically ignores the inert PEGs so when PEGs are attached to other molecules (such as interferon) the molecules stay in your system longer before your body eliminates them.

Currently, doctors are studying two PEG interferons of different lengths and molecular weights. One interferon uses a PEG of 12,000 molecular weight (PEG-INTRON™, FDA-approved in January 2001 as monotherapy, by Schering-Plough), and the other uses a PEG of 40,000 molecular weight (PEGASYS®, awaiting FDA approval as of this writing, by Roche). The interferon parts of the two PEG interferons also differ. PEGASYS® uses interferon alfa-2a, and PEG-INTRON™ uses interferon alfa-2b.

Note: Hereafter, PEG-INTRON™ will be designated in the text as Peg-Intron and PEGASYS® as Pegasys.

Pegylation is a synthetic process whereby a molecule of PEG is bonded to a molecule of interferon. Scientists precisely control the process so that the active site on the interferon molecule is not covered or damaged by the PEG molecule.

Why is pegylation important? The following discussion highlights the unique properties of pegylated interferons and their advantages over standard interferons.

Advantages of Pegylated Interferon

Because pegylation converts interferon from a relatively short-acting medication to a long-acting one by reducing the rate at which the body eliminates interferon, the time between injections is extended. Instead of three injections of standard interferon a week, the patient injects pegylated interferon only once a week.

> *I like pegylated interferon best—better than monotherapy and combo. I hated three shots a week, so it's much easier once a week.*
> *Three times a week was a roller-coaster ride, and I had three after-shot bad days. Now I have one bad day. It might be a little worse, but it's just one.*
>
> *Anna*

Pegylation makes interferon more effective in clearing hepatitis C because the addition of PEG maintains consistent and prolonged levels of interferon in the body. In contrast, non-pegylated interferons are essentially cleared within 12 to 24 hours, and injections three times a week are associated with extreme peaks and valleys of interferon levels. Patients benefit by the increased constant level of interferon, which clears hepatitis C in a greater number of cases. This advantage has been well-documented in trials comparing pegylated interferons to standard interferons (see below).

Pegylated interferon reduces the body's immune reaction to interferon. Interferons are proteins. When injected into your body, they can induce an antibody response by your immune system. In general, these antibodies have not been associated with disease, illness, or inactivation of interferon. Nonetheless, it would be best to avoid production of these antibodies, if possible. Scientists designed and directed pegylation of interferon so that it reduces the antibody reaction.

How Pegylated Interferon Works

At first, I'd start to feel the side effects 24 to 48 hours after the injection. Now, five months later, the symptoms come on in 12 hours— instant flu.

I think pegylated interferon has more residual effects than the doctors originally thought, because you're piling it up all the time.

Ray

When I tried interferon monotherapy years ago, it felt as if I had the flu, but only for a week after the first injection. It wasn't so bad after that.

Pegylated interferon is different. There's a slow buildup. It's cumulative. But I got better at compensating for the side effects.

Dan

Pegasys. The usual starting dose of Pegasys is 180 micrograms per week. The compound is pre-mixed and is in solution in a vial.

After Pegasys is injected, it slowly enters your bloodstream and takes 80 hours to reach peak concentrations in your blood. Your body slowly clears Pegasys; it takes 10 to 12 days to eliminate half of the drug. Most interferons are at least partially cleared from the body by passing through the kidneys into the urine. Pegasys is too large to be filtered by the kidneys and is not cleared by passage through the urine. Your body biodegrades the interferon and the inert 40,000 PEG passes from the liver into bile and is eliminated from your system.

Blood concentrations remain fairly constant over the course of the week between injections. With multiple doses, over the course of a year of treatment, Pegasys tends to accumulate in your body and blood levels tend to increase.

Peg-Intron. Dosage varies according to the patient's weight. For example, a 70-kilogram man who receives 1.5 micrograms per kilogram will inject 105 micrograms of Peg-Intron. The patient adds a liquid from one vial to dried powder in another and mixes the two until the powder is dissolved. The resulting solution must be injected within 24 hours.

After Peg-Intron is injected, it takes 20 hours to reach peak concentrations in your blood. Your body eliminates half a dose of Peg-Intron in two to two-and-a-half days. In contrast to Pegasys, Peg-Intron is smaller, and approximately 30 percent is cleared through the kidneys. In addition, the interferon component is biodegraded by the body, and the 12,000 molecular-weight PEG is eliminated by passage from the liver into bile and from the kidneys into urine.

There is a six-fold difference between the peak concentration and the lowest concentration achieved over the course of the week between injections. Compared to Pegasys, Peg-Intron accumulates less and has lower blood levels.

Clinical Trial Results

The following discussion is meant to provide a balanced analysis of existing trial results and is not a commercial endorsement of any given product. Our discussion of results focuses solely on intent-to-treat analyses. This means that the significance of the response is based upon all patients enrolled in the trial, not selected subgroups.

On a personal note, we realize that the following discussion is very technical and requires careful reading. Our goal has always been to translate medical jargon into everyday language without sacrificing accuracy. A full and accurate chapter on pegylated interferons presents us with the challenge of reporting on the results of multiple trials (with a voluminous amount of information) while trying to keep the text readable. I offer an analysis of the trial data at the end of each section in the hope that you find these analyses helpful in understanding pegylated interferons.

Monotherapy Trials (How Good Are Pegylated Interferons without Ribavirin?)

Pegasys. An initial study of different doses of Pegasys found that the optimal dose was 180 micrograms. This dose was evaluated in a large international multi-center study of 531 patients with chronic hepatitis C who never had prior treatment (naïve). Pegasys was compared to standard interferon (ROFERON®-A, interferon alfa-2a, Roche) over a treatment period of 48 weeks with six months of post-treatment follow-up.

Pegasys outperformed standard interferon. Sustained response, defined as undetectable HCV-RNA at six months post-treatment, was 39 percent with Pegasys and only 19 percent with standard interferon. The incremental improvement over standard interferon was 20 percent.

The sustained response in patients with genotype 1 HCV was 28 percent, compared to 7 percent in those treated with standard interferon. The spectrum of side effects observed with Pegasys was similar in frequency and severity to those observed with standard interferon. No new side effects or adverse events could be attributed to Pegasys.

Pegasys monotherapy was also evaluated in a 48-week trial of 271 patients with advanced fibrosis or compensated cirrhosis. Pegasys was significantly more effective than standard interferon in the treatment of this patient population; 30 percent of the patients who received 180 micrograms of Pegasys weekly had a sustained viral response.

In this patient population, genotype 1 HCV was relatively more resistant to treatment. Only 12 percent of patients had a sustained response.

A key question of the cirrhosis trial was to determine whether Pegasys could improve the injury and scarring (fibrosis) on liver biopsies. About two-thirds of the 271 patients in the trial had two biopsies, one before the beginning of treatment and another six months after the end of treatment. Examination of these biopsies indicated that 54 percent demonstrated improvement. Eighty-eight percent of the patients with sustained viral clearance had improved liver biopsies. In addition, a significant proportion of nonresponders (35%) also demonstrated improvement in post-treatment liver biopsies. These results suggest that Pegasys treatment may improve the degree of liver injury and scarring, not only by clearance of hepatitis C but also by a direct effect of interferon on the liver. This and similar data with other interferons were the catalyst for current and new studies, such as HALT C, that are examining the role of interferon in slowing liver injury, fibrosis, and progression of disease.

The combination therapy trial of Pegasys plus ribavirin (see below) also included a Pegasys monotherapy arm with 224 patients who were treated with 180 micrograms of Pegasys weekly for 48 weeks. The sustained response for Pegasys monotherapy in this trial was 30 percent, 21 percent for patients with genotype 1 HCV.

Peg-Intron. A large international multi-center trial examined the dosage and effectiveness of Peg-Intron compared to standard interferon (INTRON® A, interferon alfa-2b, Schering-Plough) in 1,219 patients with chronic hepatitis C, naïve to prior treatment. The Peg-Intron patients received either 0.5, 1.0, or 1.5 micrograms per kilogram of Peg-Intron for 48 weeks. The standard interferon "control group" received 3 MU three times a week for 48 weeks.

Sustained viral response was defined as undetectable for HCV-RNA six months after discontinuation of treatment. The sustained response was similar for the 1.0 and 1.5 micrograms per kilogram Peg-Intron groups (25 percent and 23 percent respectively) and superior to the sustained response for Intron A of 12 percent. Therefore, Peg-Intron was 11 to 13 percent more effective than standard interferon treatment. The sustained response for patients with genotype 1 HCV was 14 percent for Peg-Intron treatment but only 2 percent for standard interferon.

In general, the spectrum of side effects observed with Peg-Intron was similar in frequency and severity to that observed with standard interferon. No new side effects or adverse events could be attributed to Peg-Intron.

Analysis. Both pegylated interferons when given as monotherapy are more effective than standard interferon alfa-2a or standard interferon alfa-2b, and have similar side-effect profiles. For these reasons, pegylated interferons are likely to replace standard interferons, especially for patients in whom ribavirin is contraindicated.

The two pegylated interferons have not yet been compared head-to-head, and it is difficult to draw valid conclusions regarding the superiority of one over the other. However, the improved responses over standard interferon were greater for Pegasys (20 percent) than for Peg-Intron (13 percent). The greater improvement with Pegasys was also true for patients with genotype 1.

The pegylated interferons, however, may not be superior to REBE-TRON™ combination therapy [interferon alfa-2b (INTRON® A) plus ribavirin, Schering-Plough]. Reported rates of sustained response with Pegasys monotherapy range from 30 percent to 39 percent. The sustained responses in the Peg-Intron monotherapy trials ranged from 23 percent to 25 percent. These rates with pegylated interferon monotherapy are less than the reported range of sustained response for Rebetron, which is 38 percent to 47 percent.

In conclusion, pegylated interferons are superior to standard interferons as monotherapy for hepatitis C. When combination therapy is contraindicated, pegylated interferons are the treatment of choice. Existing data suggest that response is higher with Pegasys monotherapy compared to Peg-Intron monotherapy. In the future, however, most naïve patients will be treated with the combination of pegylated interferon with ribavirin. The following sections discuss the results of trials of pegylated interferons plus ribavirin.

Combination Trials (How Good Are Pegylated Interferons When Combined with Ribavirin?)

At the time of this writing, there were only two large clinical trials of the combination of pegylated interferon with ribavirin: one using Pegasys and one using Peg-Intron. We report the results of these trials in comparison to Rebetron (see Chapter 8) because Rebetron was the standard-of-care in 2001. We anticipate that pegylated interferon plus ribavirin will be the next standard-of-care. Furthermore, in our discussion we also compare the results of these two trials. Be aware that the differences reported in only two trials may not be verified once additional trials are performed.

Note: In August 2001, the FDA approved Peg-Intron for use in combination therapy with Rebetol capsules (ribavirin). Rebetol was granted FDA approval as a separately marketed product in July 2001. As of August 2001, Pegasys was awaiting FDA approval.

Pegasys. A multi-center international trial of 48 weeks evaluated the combination of Pegasys plus ribavirin. There were three arms to the study: 224 patients were treated with Pegasys monotherapy, 444 patients received Rebetron, and 453 patients were treated with Pegasys plus ribavirin. Patients in the three arms were similar in age (mean of 42 to 43 years), gender (mean of 68 to 73 percent were male), body weight (mean of 78 to 80 kilograms), genotype 1 (mean of 64 to 66 percent), and cirrhosis (mean of 12 to 15 percent).

At the end of treatment at 48 weeks, the percentages of patients that had undetectable HCV-RNA were 59 percent for Pegasys monotherapy, 52 percent for Rebetron, and 69 percent for Pegasys plus ribavirin. The increased response with Pegasys plus ribavirin was statistically significant when compared to either Pegasys monotherapy or Rebetron.

The sustained responses at six months after discontinuation of treatment were 30 percent for Pegasys monotherapy, 45 percent for Rebetron, and 56 percent for Pegasys plus ribavirin. The improved sustained response with Pegasys plus ribavirin was highly significant (P < .001) when compared to either Pegasys monotherapy or Rebetron. Pegasys plus ribavirin had an 11 percent greater sustained response than Rebetron (Figure 9A).

Sustained response to Pegasys plus ribavirin was clearly related to HCV genotype. Patients with genotype 1 had sustained responses of 21

FIGURE 9A.   SVRs with pegylated interferon plus ribavirin: all patients

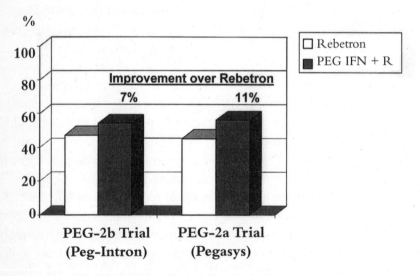

Legend 9A. The sustained viral responses (SVRs) in all patients treated for 48 weeks with either Rebetron, high-dose Peg-Intron plus ribavirin (shaded bar on left), and Pegasys plus ribavirin (shaded bar on right) are shown. In both trials, the improvement in response with pegylated interferon-based therapy (PEG IFN + R) over Rebetron was statistically significant.

percent to Pegasys monotherapy, 37 percent to Rebetron, and 46 percent to Pegasys plus ribavirin. Patients with genotypes 2 and 3 had sustained responses of 45 percent to Pegasys monotherapy, 61 percent to Rebetron, and 76 percent to Pegasys plus ribavirin. Patients with genotypes 2 or 3 were more likely than patients with genotype 1 to experience a sustained response with any of the three treatment regimens.

Results with Pegasys plus ribavirin were superior to the other two treatments for all genotypes. The 46 percent sustained response in genotype 1 patients was significantly better (P < .001) than the sustained response with either Rebetron (Figure 9B) or Pegasys monotherapy. The 76 percent sustained response in genotype 2 and 3 patients was significantly better (P < .001) than the sustained response achieved with either Rebetron or Pegasys monotherapy. One can conclude that Pegasys plus ribavirin is preferred over both Pegasys monotherapy and Rebetron.

FIGURE 9B.   SVRs WITH PEGYLATED INTERFERON PLUS
RIBAVIRIN: PATIENTS WITH GENOTYPE 1

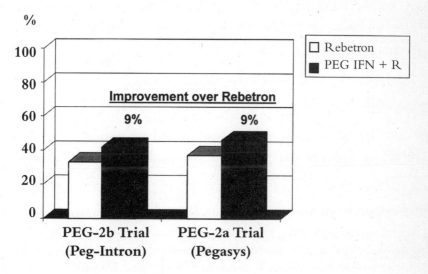

Legend 9B. The sustained responses (SVRs) in patients with genotype 1 HCV treated for 48 weeks with either Rebetron, high-dose Peg-Intron plus ribavirin (shaded bar on left), and Pegasys plus ribavirin (shaded bar on right) are shown. In both trials, the improvement in response with pegylated interferon-based therapy (PEG IFN + R) over Rebetron was statistically significant.

Side effects and rate of withdrawal from treatment with Pegasys plus ribavirin were similar to those observed with either Pegasys monotherapy or Rebetron. Patients reported a similar frequency of fatigue, headache, sleeplessness, nausea, and arthralgia (joint pains) in all three treatment arms. Fever, muscle aching, and rigors (shaking, chills) were more common with Rebetron, compared to either Pegasys monotherapy or the combination of Pegasys plus ribavirin. Thirty percent of patients in the Rebetron arm experienced depression. In contrast, only 20 percent of patients on Pegasys monotherapy and 21 percent of patients on Pegasys plus ribavirin experienced depression.

Peg-Intron. A multi-center international trial of 48 weeks evaluated the combination of Peg-Intron plus ribavirin. In this study 505 patients received Rebetron, 514 received low-dose Peg-Intron plus ribavirin, and 511 received high-dose Peg-Intron plus ribavirin. The low-dose Peg-Intron treatment consisted of Peg-Intron 1.5 micrograms per kilogram per week for four weeks followed by 0.5 micrograms per kilogram for 44 weeks plus ribavirin 1.0 to 1.2 grams per day. The high-dose Peg-Intron regimen was Peg-Intron 1.5 micrograms per kilogram per week plus ribavirin 800 milligrams per day. Patients in the three groups were similar in age (mean of 43 to 44 years), gender distribution (mean of 63 percent to 67 percent were male), body weight (mean of 82 to 83 kilograms), genotype 1 (mean of 68 percent for all three groups), and cirrhosis (mean of 10 percent for all three groups).

At the end of 48 weeks of treatment the percentages of patients that had undetectable HCV-RNA were 52 percent for Rebetron, 53 percent for low-dose Peg-Intron plus ribavirin, and 62 percent for high-dose Peg-Intron plus ribavirin. The increased viral clearance with high-dose Peg-Intron plus ribavirin was statistically significant when compared to the other two arms.

The sustained responses at six months after discontinuation of treatment were 47 percent for Rebetron, 47 percent for low-dose Peg-Intron plus ribavirin, and 54 percent for high-dose Peg-Intron plus ribavirin. The improved sustained response with high-dose Peg-Intron plus ribavirin was significant (P =.012) when compared to either Rebetron or low-dose Peg-Intron plus ribavirin. High-dose Peg-Intron plus ribavirin had a 7 percent greater sustained response than Rebetron (Figure 9A).

The likelihood of sustained response with Peg-Intron plus ribavirin was clearly related to HCV genotype. Patients with genotype 1 had sustained responses of 33 percent to Rebetron, 34 percent to low-dose Peg-

Intron plus ribavirin, and 42 percent to high-dose Peg-Intron plus rib-avirin. Patients with genotypes 2 or 3 had sustained responses of 79 per-cent to Rebetron, 80 percent to low-dose Peg-Intron plus ribavirin, and 82 percent to high-dose Peg-Intron plus ribavirin. Patients with geno-types 2 or 3 were more likely to experience sustained response with any of the three treatment regimens.

High-dose Peg-Intron plus ribavirin was superior to the other two treatments in patients with genotype 1. The 42 percent sustained response in genotype 1 patients was significantly better ($P < .001$) than the sustained response with either Rebetron (Figure 9B) or with low-dose Peg-Intron plus ribavirin. The 82 percent sustained response in genotype 2 and 3 patients was not significantly better than the sustained response achieved with either Rebetron or with low-dose Peg-Intron plus ribavirin. One can conclude that high-dose Peg-Intron plus rib-avirin is preferred over both Rebetron and low-dose Peg-Intron plus ribavirin, especially for patients with genotype 1 HCV.

Side effects of high-dose Peg-Intron plus ribavirin were similar to those observed with either Rebetron or low-dose Peg-Intron plus rib-avirin. Fever, nausea, and injection-site reactions were significantly more common with high-dose Peg-Intron plus ribavirin compared to Rebe-tron.

Analysis. Therapy using pegylated interferons with ribavirin is supe-rior to Rebetron, and has a similar side-effect profile. For these reasons, pegylated interferons plus ribavirin are likely to replace Rebetron as the treatment standard. Pegasys plus ribavirin has not yet been compared head-to-head with Peg-Intron plus ribavirin, and it is difficult to draw valid conclusions regarding the superiority of one combination over the other. However, the improvement in sustained response over Rebetron was higher for Pegasys plus ribavirin (11 percent) than for high-dose Peg-Intron plus ribavirin (7 percent) (Figure 9A).

Patients with genotype 1 experienced a higher sustained response for Pegasys plus ribavirin (46 percent) than with high-dose Peg-Intron plus ribavirin (42 percent). This difference may not be significant because the improvement over Rebetron was identical for Pegasys plus ribavirin (9 percent) and Peg-Intron plus ribavirin (9 percent) (Figure 9B).

Reported side effects with Pegasys plus ribavirin were similar to or less than those observed with Rebetron. Reported side effects with high-dose Peg-Intron plus ribavirin were similar to or higher than those observed with Rebetron.

In conclusion, the combination of pegylated interferon with ribavirin represents the next standard-of-care in the treatment of patients with chronic hepatitis C. Two current regimens, Pegasys plus ribavirin and high-dose Peg-Intron plus ribavirin, are superior to Rebetron. Sustained response, side-effect profile, cost, ease of administration, compliance with treatment, and patient and physician preference may ultimately determine which regimen is used in a given patient.

The Patient's Experience: Treatment with Pegylated Interferon Plus Ribavirin

Note: Please refer to The Patient's Experience in Chapter 8 for information about injections and the side effects of both interferon and ribavirin. Note also that each person reacts differently to treatment.

With my first dose, I had the worst side effects ever. My teeth were chattering, and I had a fever. But by the next week, it wasn't as bad.

Although I had a lot of the same side effects I had when I took combination therapy, everything started improving after I learned I was virus-free! My hair doesn't come out in handfuls anymore. Body aches are down, and the fatigue is a little better.

The first dose was not as bad as regular interferon. I compare myself to others who are really sick, or so tired they can't do anything. It didn't make me feel like that.

I take my shot on Monday night. On Tuesday or Wednesday, I get the reaction: a temperature, achy muscles. I take Tylenol®, and by the next morning I'm fine.

When I took the first dose, I got chills and nausea. I went into work, and I started shaking. My teeth were chattering. I had the sweats. I missed three days of work, so I called the nurse and said I can't handle this. I can't miss work.

The nurse was a big help. She encouraged me. After the second shot, my body got used to it. But I didn't like having dry, itchy skin, especially around the injection areas, and the tiredness and depression. I felt like a martyr.

Why did I stick with it? I try to keep my word. If I tell someone I'm going to do something, I do it.

And a year later, my blood tests show that the virus is still undetectable!

I'd get tired if I carried groceries from the car to the house. The doctor thought that maybe I'd have to cut back on work, but I never did. Treatment did not interfere with my work, daily functions, or my family at all.

It's unbelievable to deal with your emotions. Every week they mutate, like the virus. Every week is different.

I have a blue-collar mentality. My dad always said a little hard work never killed anybody. So when I can't go out and do stuff, I feel bad.

The sprinkler broke. I got all my tools out. Where do you think they all are two months later? Still in the same place! I had to fix the pump or the lawn would die, but I had no energy, no will to put the tools back. It's a mental thing.

I call it "the day-after-the-shot day." It's pretty dramatic. That's when I have most of my body aches and pains. I can't function. I go to bed after work at 5 o'clock. I'm doing better now; I can stay up until 8.

I started at a high dose, but it was reduced because of my blood counts. The treatment wasn't agreeing with me, but I had no side effects, no fatigue, no weight loss. The only thing I can recall was the itching that started around six months. No rash—but I'd itch like crazy on the lower part of my ankles, legs, and the back of my neck.

The hardest part was trying to communicate what treatment is like to my family and friends. I had a hard time with that—with getting them to understand that I can't go out, that I'm exhausted and it wouldn't be any fun.

I've had hepatitis C for 30 years, and I think their attitude is, "What's new? Why are you whining?"

I responded. That was the wonderful part. I didn't expect it after other courses of therapy and a diagnosis of cirrhosis. Then I got a rash so bad, I had to quit taking ribavirin. It was all over my body—even in my mouth—and so painful I couldn't sleep.

I thought that without ribavirin, pegylated interferon alone wouldn't clear the virus. But it did!

I'd have a red spot where I injected the needle for a few days after the injection. Then it would go away. Over the year, the red spots turned black. I'd have black marks on my thighs. I refused to wear shorts. Two to three months after I was done with treatment, they totally went away.

I didn't go to church for six months. I just slept. It's a miracle I didn't lose my business. God had His hand in it.

Pegylated? It was Greek to me when I started. You get an education as you go. I was very optimistic, glad to have hope.

I felt blessed. That's as good a word as any. I never felt I was particularly deserving of anything special. Why was I picked to be someone who responded?

I'm the head of a national sales force. A lot of people were depending on me to keep them from being laid off when the company went through a period of turmoil while I was on treatment. I felt like a shepherd with a flock. I couldn't let them down. Maybe that's why I got the extra strength.

I didn't clear the virus, but a recent biopsy showed that the inflammation and fibrosis improved. My liver went from stage II back to stage I.

Myalgia kept me awake. I had this gnawing, irritating grinding in my muscles. The doctor put me on sleep medicine. I was so desperate for sleep.

It worked, and with no hangover, too. It just shut my mind off so I only took it at home. I had no problem getting off it after treatment.

I said, "Well, okay, I did not respond to the medicine. But it's not over yet because the Great Physician—God—is still at work, and I am not giving up." I refuse to believe that I will have to live the rest of my life with this virus inside me.

I didn't think regular interferon was a big deal. I wouldn't say that about pegylated interferon and ribavirin, but I've never gotten to the point where I can't function.

I filled out this form that asked me if I felt good or bad. I don't feel either. My sexual desire is gone. I feel like a machine. I do things because I have to do them.

The first test showed I was responding. Anybody who is going to take this treatment has to be committed. I've thought about quitting, but giving up would be worse. I've had hepatitis C since 1988, and I want to get rid of it.

Treatment made me more compassionate. I used to avoid people who were suffering from other diseases because I didn't know what to say. Now I go right up to them, and I ask them how they're REALLY doing.

Treatment Tips from Patients on Pegylated Interferon Plus Ribavirin

Note: See Treatment Tips in Chapter 8 for additional suggestions.

I call it my bath therapy—soaking in a tub with mineral salts. It really helps me relax.

I try not to think about the side effects. I look at the end result and keep my eyes on the prize.

I had to rearrange my thinking around an emotional, mental wall. I hadn't talked to anyone until I confided in a friend who had cancer and chemotherapy. I'm lucky I picked him because he knows exactly what I'm going through.

Once I found out I was in remission, there was hope. So I finally told my dad.

If I walk up a flight of stairs, I'm huffing and puffing because ribavirin lowers your oxygen. I have to stop on the landing and take deep breaths to get more air into my system.

I try very hard to take a nap in my car at lunchtime. It helps me get through the workday.

I work full time. I was raised to think that when you quit, that's when you die. So you just keep going. When both my white and red blood counts dropped, I was doing what I had to do, but I was in a total fog. My boss said, "You're going to have to start writing things down."

The doctors reduced my doses of both interferon and ribavirin and I went on an antidepressant. That helped.

I took baths in an Aveeno® bath treatment with oatmeal powder for the itching, and I used their anti-itch cream, too.

Baking soda and water worked as well as anything for the itching.

I'm exhausted all the time. I go to bed at 7 o'clock at night and get up at 7 o'clock in the morning. I'm rarely up to see the sunset.

Exercise helps. At first I got tired, but now I'm doing better. I started with 9 holes of golf, and I've worked my way up to 18.

I run out of gas, and I feel spaced out. I enjoy a nap now and then.

I never missed a day of work. I took the meds with me when I had to travel, icing them down.

I'd also time my shots. I started on Friday, and I'd have 36 hours with aches, pains, and headaches. By the time Monday came, I was feeling alright to work. I could do routine stuff. By Wednesday I was feeling like myself again. I would plan complicated projects on Thursday and Friday when I was mentally sharper.

I was always cold. It felt like I stayed cold for the whole 48 weeks of treatment. I never put on shorts that year. Instead, I wore insulated jeans.

I drink a lot of water. I have water bottles everywhere, at home, at work. I never drink pop. I only drink filtered water.

I don't concentrate as well on this interferon so I use a hand-held computer. I set it to buzz me when it's time to take the ribavirin. Then on the screen it asks me if I took it, and I have to insert "yes." I've never missed any ribavirin or injections.

I'd get redness at the site of the injection, but I learned to rotate the injection sites, move the needle around. The redness went away after a couple of months.

My faith and spirituality help me through it. I have wonderful church support with people praying for my healing.

One day at a time. I never understood that saying until the doctor told me I only had five years left. Okay, I thought. I'd better take that cruise now. When I think of something I always wanted to do and I can afford it, I do it now. I even went parasailing last May!

I look at it this way. The rash is ugly, but the fact that I have it means that at least my body knows something is going on!

I'm very conscious of what I eat. I cut back on sweets, junk food, and I eat a lot of fruit with fiber. I also drink lots of water and apple, cran-berry, and orange juice. I even juice my own apples and veggies.

Treatment of Nonresponders or Relapsers (What Are Your Chances of Responding to Pegylated Interferons Plus Ribavirin?)

If the prior therapy failed to clear the virus (nonresponse), or the virus returned in your blood after initial clearance (relapse), then re-treatment with the combination of pegylated interferon plus ribavirin should be considered. Relapse is not the same as nonresponse. In patients who relapse, the virus is undetectable during the course of treatment, but resurfaces after treatment ends. Nonresponse means that the virus was detectable throughout the course of treatment. Relapse is common with interferon monotherapy but less common with Rebetron or pegylated interferon plus ribavirin.

Nonresponse or relapse occurs for five main reasons:

1. The therapy used was ineffective.
2. The patient did not comply with prescribed treatment.
3. Treatment doses had to be reduced due to low levels of white cells, red cells, or platelets.
4. Length of treatment or dose was reduced due to side effects or poor quality of life.
5. The type of hepatitis C infection was relatively or absolutely resistant to interferon-based treatment.

Projected Results with Re-Treatment: Can We Peer into the Future? If you received prior therapy, you may ask the question, "Does it make any sense to be re-treated?" Any patient who failed to clear hepatitis C on any previous treatment regimen is potentially a candidate for re-treatment with the combination of pegylated interferon plus ribavirin.

My first treatment was just interferon, not the cocktail. It was a piece of cake. I seemed to adjust in a month-and-a-half, but I lost my response. I relapsed. And then I went into denial. I thought maybe my symptoms were a weird residual thing left over from the malaria I had in the army.

After several years of depression and putting hepatitis C on the back burner, I started to get a dull ache in my liver area. I decided that I needed to get proactive and understand the disease. When my doctor told me I might qualify for a study of pegylated interferon, I went for it because I don't have any health insurance.

Actually, the first time I took interferon was not a piece of cake, but the pegylated interferon with ribavirin was much harder. It got my attention. But I trained myself to be very positive.

At the end of the month, I told my nurse that my blood tests were going to be normal. She said that would be unusual. A few days later, she called with the results. They were normal!

Tom

At the time of this writing, patients should consider re-treatment if they previously failed to clear the virus with interferon monotherapy, pegylated interferon monotherapy, Rebetron, or sub-optimal doses of peginterferon plus ribavirin. More data will emerge in the next one to three years regarding the success of re-treatment using pegylated interferon plus ribavirin.

The predicted responses to re-treatment, according to the type of prior therapy and HCV genotype, are shown in Table 9A. For all patients, re-treatment with the combination of pegylated interferon plus ribavirin may lead to viral clearance in approximately 50 percent of those who failed interferon monotherapy. The chance for a sustained response is 18 to 35 percent for those who failed Rebetron and 27 to 40 percent for those who failed monotherapy with one of the pegylated interferons. Patients with HCV genotype 1 are less likely than patients with genotype 2 or 3 to respond (see Table 9A).

When faced with the decision to re-treat, most physicians will recommend the combination of pegylated interferon plus ribavirin. In my opinion, nonresponders and relapsers to interferon monotherapy, pegylated interferon monotherapy, and Rebetron have a reasonable chance to clear hepatitis C with re-treatment with pegylated interferon plus ribavirin and should be given the opportunity.

Alternatives to Pegylated Interferons Plus Ribavirin

Pegylated interferon plus ribavirin is emerging as the preferred treatment for patients with hepatitis C. However, there may be medical or other reasons why your doctor may not prescribe this treatment. Certain underlying conditions, such as renal (kidney) failure, dialysis, anemia, and use of medications that impair kidney function (cyclosporine, tacrolimus), may contraindicate the use of ribavirin. In the latter circumstances, pegylated interferon as monotherapy might be preferred over ribavirin-based combinations.

If pegylated interferon plus ribavirin is not available, your physician may recommend either Rebetron or pegylated interferon monotherapy. The results will be less than expected with the combination of pegylated interferon plus ribavirin but still may result in a viral cure in a significant percentage of cases.

Another unresolved issue is whether the long-term use of ribavirin in women of childbearing age is safe in terms of outcomes of subsequent

TABLE 9A: PREDICTED RATES OF SUSTAINED RESPONSE AFTER RE-TREATMENT WITH PEGYLATED INTERFERON PLUS RIBAVIRIN

Prior Antiviral Therapy	Predicted Sustained Response (%) after Re-Treatment with Peginterferon plus Ribavirin	
	Patients with Genotype	
	1	2 & 3
Interferon, tiw, 6 months	41%	75%
Interferon, tiw, 12 months	38%	70%
REBETRON, 6 months	31%	32%
REBETRON, 12 months	8 to 19%	14 to 38%
PEGASYS monotherapy, 12 months	19 to 34%	60%
PEG-INTRON monotherapy, 12 months	33%	60%

This table depicts the expected rates of response to re-treatment of nonresponders with 48 weeks of pegylated interferon plus ribavirin. The spectrum of nonresponders includes those who failed to clear HCV after short-term or long-term treatment with either interferon monotherapy or Rebetron or those who failed 12 months of monotherapy with pegylated interferons.

Response rates for re-treatment were calculated from the equation: % Sustained Response = $[(SR_{PEG+R} \% - SR_{Rx1} \%)/(100\% - SR_{Rx1} \%)]$ x 100%. The sustained response (SR_{PEG+R} %) used for patients with genotype 1 HCV was 44%, the average of the results in the Pegasys (46%) and Peg-Intron (42%) trials. The sustained response (SR_{PEG+R} %) used for patients with genotypes 2 & 3 was 79%, the average of the results in the Pegasys (76%) and Peg-Intron (82%) trials, except for the situation where the initial treatment was 12 months of Rebetron. In the latter circumstance, data was compared within trial. In the Pegasys trial the response to Pegasys plus ribavirin was 76% and the response to Rebetron, 61%. In the Peg-Intron trial the response to Peg-Intron plus ribavirin was 82% and the response to Rebetron, 79%.

SR_{Rx1} % was the sustained response rate that could have been achieved with the prior therapy as reported in the medical literature. The SR_{Rx1} % for patients with genotype 1 HCV for each of the treatments were: interferon, tiw, 6 months, pregnancies. Clearly, use of ribavirin during pregnancy is contraindicated, and appropriate and effective methods of contraception must be practiced during and for at least six months after any course of treatment containing ribavirin. Nonetheless, pregnancies have occurred in women taking ribavirin, and these pregnancies have been characterized by a high rate of miscarriage and occasional chromosomal abnormalities and birth defects. It is not known whether pregnancies that occur six months and beyond completion of treatment are complicated by either miscarriage or birth defects. Perhaps pegylated interferon monotherapy has a place in the initial treatment of women of childbearing age.

In summary, I am very excited by the current results of studies using pegylated interferon with ribavirin. Today more than 50 percent of patients with hepatitis C may be cured of their infection. In my opinion, pegylated interferon with ribavirin is the emerging standard-of-care in the treatment of hepatitis C.

> *No physician, insofar as he is a physician, considers his own good in what he prescribes, but the good of his patient.*
>
> *Plato*

2%; interferon, tiw, 12 months, 7%; Rebetron, 6 months, 16%; Rebetron, 12 months, 28% to 37%; Pegasys monotherapy, 12 months, 12% to 28%; and Peg-Intron monotherapy, 12 months, 14%. The SR$_{Rxt}$ % for patients with genotypes 2 & 3 for each of the treatments were: interferon, tiw, 6 months, 16%; interferon, tiw, 12 months, 29%; Rebetron, 6 months, 69%; Rebetron, 12 months, 61% (Pegasys trial) to 79% (Peg-Intron trial); Pegasys monotherapy, 12 months, 48% (average of results from the monotherapy arm of the Pegasys plus ribavirin trial (45%), and the results of the Pegasys cirrhosis trial (51%); and Peg-Intron monotherapy, 12 months, 48% (average for 1.0 ug/kg (47%)and 1.5 ug/kg (49%) arms of trial). The calculation of re-treatment response for those initially treated with 12 months of Rebetron was trial specific (see above).

Please note that the sustained response rates reported in this table were derived from existing literature describing the treatment of naïve patients. The response rates for nonresponders listed in the table have not yet been verified by properly controlled clinical trials.

Reference

1. The Hepatitis C Antiviral Long-Term Treatment Against Cirrhosis (HALT C) is the NIH-sponsored clinical trial of the use of Pegasys plus ribavirin in the treatment of nonresponders to prior therapy.

1 0

LIVER TRANSPLANTS
A Miracle of Modern Medicine

I was on the liver transplant waiting list for—oh, gosh—nine months. Finally, they gave me a pager because it was getting close. The second day, early in the morning, I was sleeping in that ozone where you're just starting to wake up, when I heard the pager go off. I bolted out of bed. I hadn't moved like that for months because I'd been so sick.

I reached for my pager, but it wasn't blinking. My heart was just pounding! Then I heard the garbage truck in the alley; it was the warning beep as the truck backed up.

The real call came three weeks later at 4:30 a.m. The doctors kept asking me if I was afraid, if I was sure I wanted to do this. "My God, yes!" I said. "Let's get this show on the road."

Tom

SOME PEOPLE WITH HEPATITIS C develop cirrhosis, liver failure, and need a liver transplant to survive. Liver transplantation is the most complicated therapy for people with end-stage hepatitis C, but it can produce seemingly miraculous results.

Pre-transplant patients go through a difficult time. They suffer from a variety of symptoms, including jaundice, sleeplessness, itching, fluid buildup, mental confusion, and hemorrhaging. A successful transplant cures these symptoms, and the patient can lead a full, productive life.

This chapter covers the following topics:

Liver Transplantation: A Brief History

The first liver transplant was performed by Dr. Thomas Starzl in 1963 at the University of Colorado in Denver. Twenty years later, in 1983, a National Institutes of Health (NIH) consensus conference on the therapeutic role of liver transplantation concluded, "After extensive review and consideration…liver transplantation is a therapeutic modality for end-stage liver disease that deserves broader application."

At that time, only six centers in North America and four in Europe performed liver transplantation. Ten years later, 3,442 patients had the procedure at 88 centers in the United States. As of July 6, 2001, there were 18,028 patients on the active U.S. waiting list.

Who Gets a Liver Transplant?

The Most Common Diagnosis: Hepatitis C. Liver transplantation is the most successful therapy for patients with a wide array of diseases that ultimately result in liver failure. Currently, the most common diagnosis for transplant is cirrhosis due to chronic hepatitis C. Laennec's cirrhosis, caused by alcohol, ranks second, but co-infection with hepatitis C is common in these patients—illustrating once again that the combination of alcohol and hepatitis C speeds the progression of liver disease.

Signs That You Need a Transplant. Obvious clinical signs and symptoms usually accompany advanced liver disease, including:

- ascites (accumulation of fluid in the abdomen)
- encephalopathy (alteration of mental function)
- variceal hemorrhage (bleeding from veins in the esophagus or stomach)
- worsening nutritional status
- diminishing quality of life

Patients who have a spontaneous infection in the ascites fluid, low serum albumin (< 2.8 grams/deciliter), clotting problems (prothrombin time > 5 seconds prolonged), and severe sustained jaundice should be given urgent consideration for transplantation. All of the above findings indicate severe liver dysfunction and are late signs of end-stage liver disease.

> *I found out I had hepatitis C when I came to the hospital a year ago. I had a lot of fluid in my stomach. They drained me and sent me home. I couldn't sleep. I'd lay down, stand up. The only way I could get some sleep was to fill the bathtub up so I could get some buoyancy, which relieved the pain in my stomach.*
>
> *The second time I had to go to the hospital, they did an ultrasound. That's how I found out I needed a transplant.*
>
> Chris

Many people with cirrhosis have few or no findings of liver disease. Doctors say that these patients have "compensated" cirrhosis, and that it may be too early to consider liver transplantation. However, the waiting list for liver transplants is expanding, while the pool of donors is staying about the same. Patients often wait on the list for one, two, or more years before they get a liver.

Once you have cirrhosis, your doctor must monitor your blood tests closely and watch for any physical signs of decompensation in order to time the referral for liver transplantation. Unfortunately, not all patients with compensated cirrhosis are the same; some will remain stable for several years, but others may deteriorate relatively rapidly.

The course of hepatitis C varies greatly, so your physician must make an imperfect estimate of your chances of having a life-threatening complication over a one- to two-year follow-up period. If your doctor estimates that you have more than a 10 percent chance of sustaining a complication within one year, you should be evaluated for transplantation.

Denial of Transplants. You may be denied a liver transplant if you have active HIV infection or AIDS, incurable cancer, active infection in the blood, active alcohol abuse, or severe underlying heart, lung, or multi-organ disease. If you are elderly, morbidly obese, or have had prior extensive abdominal surgery, a clotted portal vein, extensive liver cancer, an isolated liver cancer larger than five centimeters, or cancer of the bile ducts, you might be excluded from transplantation.

Paying for Transplants. See Chapter 7, Taking Care of Yourself Financially.

The Transplant Team

Liver transplantation is a complex procedure requiring many specialists to care for you. Usually, your transplant team consists of a hepatologist, a hepatology nurse, a transplant surgeon, a transplant anesthesiologist, a transplant nurse coordinator (who keeps you informed and tells you when a liver becomes available), a social worker (who provides you and your family with emotional support), a psychiatrist (who meets with you and your family to evaluate your strengths and weaknesses and make recommendations to help you through the transplant experience), a nutritionist (who deals with pre-transplant issues, such as overweight problems or nutritional wasting, and helps with recommendations for your post-transplant nutritional needs), and a financial coordinator. Your outcome is improved if your liver transplant program has a "team" approach and performs more than 20 transplants a year.

Waiting for a Liver

The Evaluation Process. You will be asked to take many diagnostic tests and meet with a psychiatrist and social worker. Usually, you meet with each person on the transplant team. The process can take a couple of days. When all the tests and interviews are completed, the team meets to approve or deny your candidacy for transplantation and may suggest additional evaluations or consultations.

> *I had two days of evaluation, from early morning until 5 o'clock in the evening. The tests were tough, but I got a lot of kindness and attention. I met everybody—the psychiatrist, the surgical team. I had to bring my whole family to the social worker. Oh boy, I've never had such tests. At my first stop, they took 21 vials of blood!*
>
> *They were very frank with me. They wouldn't waste a liver if other things were wrong with me. My previous doctor had told me I was too old to get a liver. I'm 61. The transplant team said I checked out to be in pretty good health for my age, and now I'm on the waiting list.*
>
> *Carla*

> *At my evaluation, the psychiatrist must have asked me ten times if I was a closet drinker. I know they have to find out if you're an active alcoholic, but I found it offensive. Everyone assumes that you're an alcoholic if you need a liver transplant. That's the first thing you have to overcome.*
>
> *Bea*

> *When they asked me why I thought I should get a transplant, I said, "I have seven grandchildren. I have much to teach and share. When I get my liver, as soon as I'm able, I intend to educate people and speak to people about becoming donors."*
>
> *Leonora*

In trying to evaluate your ability to tolerate transplant surgery, the transplant team will give you some diagnostic tests. Depending on your condition, the tests may include blood tests, colonoscopy (view of the entire colon through a colonoscope), CT scan (a radiologic test that lets doctors see the anatomy and size of your liver), ECG (an electrocardio-gram), endoscopy (a procedure that allows doctors to look for ulcers, masses, varices, or bleeding in the esophagus or stomach), ERCP (a pro-cedure performed when there is concern about blockage or narrowing in the bile ducts), flexible sigmoidoscopy (a procedure that lets the physician look at the lower colon for polyps, hemorrhoids, ulcers, and colon or rectal cancer), pulmonary function tests (a breathing test that measures the function of your lungs), and ultrasound (a test that gives information about the size and shape of your liver through sound waves). If you have conditions that require additional tests, you may be asked to meet with a consultant, such as a cardiologist.

The Waiting List. As previously noted, the number of patients on the waiting list continues to expand. Current patients placed on the list can wait for more than two years for a donor liver. This is an incredibly difficult and apprehensive period. While waiting, you may have to deal with life changes, physical symptoms, and financial changes. If you're the major breadwinner who can't go to work, you may lose the social net-work from your job.

> *Life is on hold. I haven't had too many problems, except mentally—I worry a lot. The toxins make your mind goofy. I can't remember things or make good judgments.*
>
> *And it's hard on my wife. This mental problem has been developing over years, and we didn't know why, so we've had a lot of marital prob-lems. We go to counseling, and we've learned to fight fair, but she's scared of the hepatitis C. She doesn't have any desire to be intimate with me at all. It's pretty hard.*
>
> *It's hard for me to accept knowing that I'm dying. I only have 10 to 15 percent usage of my liver. I've been in and out of the hospital five times. Sometimes I wonder if I'll die before I get a liver.*
>
> *Thomas*

I've been on the waiting list for seven months. It's like an out-of-body experience—as if it's happening to someone else, not to me. Sometimes I realize I have lots to get in order, because a percentage of people don't make it. You want a liver to come, and yet you don't.

Normally, I can battle the depression, but last night I couldn't sleep. I tossed and turned. When that happens, I start cooking. I love to cook.

Johanna

I waited 515 days for my liver—and each day was a little more painful and difficult than the day before.

I think the secret of my success during surgery was maintaining a positive attitude. I packed my suitcase in August with a red flannel robe and a Santa Claus hat. It was hot, and I felt lousy, so why did I pack for Christmas?

I was baking Christmas cookies with my grandchildren when the phone rang. Laughing and covered from head to toe in flour, I asked my husband to tell whoever it was that I was too busy for a transplant. It was the call from the hospital. I got my liver that night.

Deanne

A diminishing number of patients are transplanted in stable condition from home [United Network for Organ Sharing (UNOS) status 3]. From January 1997 to July 2001 at the University of Colorado program we performed 350 transplants, and only a few were done in patients at UNOS status 3. Increasingly, transplants are performed in sicker patients who are hospitalized or in intensive care.

It's critical at this stage to talk about your struggles with a good friend or therapist. Keeping a personal journal is helpful. You are going through a fundamental shift in how you think of yourself and preparing for the psychological changes of the transplant.

Transplant Support Groups. Transplant support groups can be a source of strength and encouragement for pre- and post-transplant patients. The long waiting period, difficult symptoms, the trauma of surgery, the psychological shift of accepting another person's organ—all of these issues are unique to transplant patients. No one else can truly understand what it's like.

I feel a lot more comfortable in the support group now than I did six months ago. Getting to know the people, being involved with their lives, and caring for each other have helped.

When people get their transplants, it's like day and night. I look at myself as night, and they're day. Sam, he just got his. I watched him go through his struggle, and he looked really bad. It's amazing what a new liver can do for a person. It's a shot in the arm. Their facial expressions change. They glow.

I feel happier, less depressed. I don't participate a lot in the group, but I'm learning. When I get my transplant, I'll go to the group because it seems to be a help to new people who come in.

The tiredness, not sleeping, itching—no one else can know how bad you feel. They wouldn't believe it if you told them. You need to talk, to vent. If I talked to my family, I'd cry and they'd cry. You don't need that. How you feel is how you feel.

It helped me to see others waiting. I was a basket case, but I began to accept that it was going to happen. I'd get my liver.

I cried at the group the first time I went. To see all those people—it was overwhelming. For the first time, my husband felt positive about the transplant. He had been reluctant to have me go through it, but he saw so many people looking so good and doing so well.

I think everyone should be required to go to a transplant support group. At first I dug my heels in and refused to go. I had the feeling I was assisting Mother Nature and wondered whether I had the right to do that. When I saw others in the support group, I decided if I could have that quality of life back, I'd go for it.

Your transplant team can refer you to a support group, or you can check the resources listed at the end of this chapter. In addition to support groups, many people tell me they find it helpful to read about other liver transplant patients' experiences and about the procedure itself. Here are some books my patients recommend:

Resources:

Green, Reg. *The Nicholas Effect, A Boy's Gift to the World*. Sepastopol: O'Reilly, 1999.

Maier, Frank with Ginny Maier. *Sweet Reprieve*. New York: Crown, 1991.

McCartney, Scott. *Defying the Gods*. New York: Macmillan, 1994.

Schomaker, Mary Zimmeth. *Life Line, How One Night Changed Five Lives*. Far Hills: New Horizon, 1996.

Starzl, Thomas E. *The Puzzle People*. Pittsburgh: University of Pittsburgh, 1992.

Liver Transplant Surgery

Donor Livers. Liver transplantation is made possible only through the act of organ donation. In most states, you can sign an organ donor permission statement on your driver's license; a witnessed signature is a legal form of consent. Most organ procurement organizations, however, request additional consent from the closest living relative. These organizations identify potential donors by interacting with emergency rooms and intensive care units.

Organ donation is one of the highest forms of giving and caring, and the vast majority of religious denominations endorse it. The generosity of organ donation makes possible the miracle of transplantation. Here is Judy Ferrin's story:

> At the hospital, the doctors diagnosed my daughter, Allison, with toxic shock syndrome. She went from laughing and joking with me to sleeping, a coma, and dying within 24 hours. She was 19 years old.
>
> Just three weeks before, the two of us were watching a little boy on TV who needed a new heart. We decided to donate our organs if something happened to us—so I knew what her wishes were, and I told her nurse.
>
> The night before the funeral, I tossed and turned. I felt a need to speak at the service, but I was so afraid. We got a call from the doctor that morning. They had successfully transplanted her kidneys. Other organs were also transplanted, but that was the first, the turning point. A wave of relief went over me. And I was able to speak about Allison to the hundreds of people who came to mourn with our family.
>
> When we give to other people, it helps us through our grief. It helps us as much as the people we give to.

Did you know that the liver donor usually donates as many as seven organs for seven different patients? Suitable liver donors are patients under age 65 who are brain-dead but whose hearts are beating. (In some cases, donors as old as 80 have been used.) They have no underlying malignancy, and they test negative for AIDS and active hepatitis B. The donors must have stable heart function with acceptable liver tests, serum sodium less than 170, and preferably been hospitalized for fewer than seven days. Donors and recipients must have compatible blood types and approximately similar body size but not identical gender.

It's customary to biopsy the donor liver to be certain that it is not scarred, fatty, or severely damaged. Once recovered, the donated organs are flushed with a special solution that preserves them for up to 48 hours.

Patients frequently ask whether organs from donors who test positive for hepatitis C can be used for transplantation. Yes, but the recipient will acquire hepatitis C. One study followed 29 recipients of organs from 13 donors who tested positive for hepatitis C. Twenty-eight of the 29 recipients tested positive for hepatitis C after the transplant. For this reason, we restrict the use of these donor livers to recipients who already have hepatitis C or who are critically ill. The latter patients need urgent transplantation and are listed at high UNOS status. (For more information on UNOS, see Resources at the end of this chapter.)

Despite efforts to use all potential donor organs, we currently face a crisis in supply and availability of donor organs. We encourage all readers of this book to work with their local organ procurement organizations to increase public awareness of the critical need and value of organ donation. It's important for all family members to discuss organ and tissue donation. Everyone should consider signing a Uniform Donor Card.

Resource: For more information on organ donation, contact the Coalition on Donation, an alliance of national organizations and local coalitions that educates the public about organ donation at 804-330-8620; email: coalition@unos.org; website: www.shareyourlife.org.

How can physicians attempt to deal with the crisis in availability of donor organs? The cadaveric supply of donor livers has remained relatively constant at about 4,000 to 4,500 donor livers each year for the past five years. The current U.S. waiting list is over 16,000.

We need to increase the donor pool in innovative ways in order to meet the expanding need for donor organs. Use of older donors, livers with increased amounts of fat, and hepatitis C antibody-positive livers has failed to substantially expand the donor pool. Splitting of cadaveric livers for use in two recipients works well for a pediatric (left lateral segment) and adult recipient (right lobe + left medial segment); splits for two adult recipients works less well. For this reason, our center and many others have embarked upon the use of adult living donors (right lobe donation) for adults.

Living-Donor Liver Transplant. You may be thinking, "By the time I need a transplant, there will be too many people on the waiting list, and I won't ever get one!" One solution for the shortage of donors may be living-donor liver transplantation, where a portion of a living donor's liver is removed and then transplanted. The Japanese, for example, still debate the concept of brain death so most liver donations in Japan are from live donors. In the past, the majority of live donor transplant operations were performed in pediatric recipients. Currently in the U.S., however, more live donor liver transplants are performed in adult than pediatric recipients.

At the time of this writing, the University of Colorado has performed more than 50 adult-to-adult live-donor liver transplantions with the vast majority between relatives, although close friends and personal relationships may be considered. All donors are alive and tolerated the liver resection. Their livers regenerated back to normal size within 16 weeks.

We recently evaluated the impact of right lobe donation on the quality of life of the living donors:

- 75 percent of donors recovered completely and returned to normal life within an average of 3.4 months after surgery.
- 96 percent returned to work at an average of 2.4 months.
- 42 percent described a change in body image related to the scar from the incision.
- 71 percent had mild ongoing abdominal discomfort.

Personal relationships between donor and recipient were the same or better in 96 percent of cases. The relationship of the donor to his or her life partner was the same or better in 80 percent of cases. Most donors reported out-of-pocket expenses not covered by insurance plans. All patients reported that under the same circumstances they would donate again, and 96 percent of the donors felt that they benefited from the experience.

Survival and rates of retransplantation in recipients of living-donor liver transplants are similar to results after cadaveric transplants. Biliary complications occur more frequently compared to standard cadaveric transplantation. However, because of the critical lack of cadaveric donor livers, it is my opinion that living-donor donation for adults will become increasingly common in the United States.

In our program, we have developed selection criteria for both donor and recipient. Our current criteria for selection of recipients center around two concepts. First, we feel that recipients should have an excellent chance for favorable post-transplant outcome. Second, the recipient should be in urgent need of a transplant for survival and might die while waiting for standard cadaveric transplantation.

Donors for living-donor liver transplantation must be relatively young (less than 50 years old), normal body size, healthy without medical problems, and they cannot have a history of prior abdominal surgery. Donors and recipients should have compatible blood types and an emotional bond. Unlike other transplants, livers do not need to be matched by tissue type. The donor liver, however, must be of sufficient size that a lobe will be large enough for the recipient.

In 1997 Karen Frederick had been fighting for her life for 14 long months on the liver transplant waiting list. Her older sister, Christine Larsen, was a little taller, bigger, and had the same blood type:

Karen's skin was gray. Her mind was gone. She couldn't walk or make a sentence. She didn't know who people were. She knew me on occasion, but she'd fade in and out.

Christine

I had to have a transplant, so I came to terms with it. But if anything happened to my sister, I don't know if I could live with it. My doctor said I had to accept that it was her decision.

Karen

After the operation, we lived in the same hospital room for seven days. Later we learned the doctors felt the sibling rivalry would make us get better quicker. They were right. We got into who could blowcomb their hair sooner, faster, better.

Christine

We prepared for our hospital stay by buying matching T-shirts with funny faces and boxer shorts.

Karen

I was surprised. Even the first day after the operation, she was making more sense. She lost that gray color.

Christine

I got her right lobe. They told us it would take six weeks for both of our livers to grow back to normal size. Ten days after the operation, Christine was leaving to go home. On our way to the airport, we stopped at the hospital for CT scans. And we both had full-sized livers!

Karen

I love coffee ice cream, and Karen never did until after the transplant. "Look what you've done," she tells me.
I love cilantro. She hates it. When she starts to eat cilantro, I'll know that the livers are in perfect shape!

Christine

At the airport, when Christine was going home, I was tearful. "I can never thank you enough," I said. Then I gave her a quick hug and zoom, we were off. Neither of us is big on mushy stuff. But she knows how I feel.

Karen

The living donor undergoes careful medical, psychological, and social evaluation. Potential donors may be rejected because their livers are unsuitable or they have underlying medical conditions that increase the risk of complications from surgery.

Risk to the donor is small but present. The current estimate of the risk of death is 1 in 500 liver donations. Other complications can occur, however, including pulmonary emboli, gastrointestinal bleeding, bile duct injury, bile leak, and infection. The overall rate of serious complications in donors is approximately 10 percent. The liver is the only internal human organ that regenerates itself; the portion of the liver that is removed regenerates over 8 to 16 weeks.

The overall outcome for recipients primarily relates to their pretransplant clinical condition. When the procedure is performed in stable patients under non-urgent conditions, the one-year survival rate is greater than 90 percent. Survival rates decrease when the transplant takes place in more urgent circumstances. It is likely that living-donor liver transplantation will become commonplace in the future, and selection criteria will change.

The Surgical Procedure. The human body has two kidneys, two lungs—but only one liver. Scientists have created artificial kidneys (kidney dialysis) and even artificial hearts, but no one has been able to duplicate the hundreds of functions of the liver to create an effective liver dialysis machine. Liver transplant surgery, therefore, has no fall-back position, no margin for error.

Although the original method pioneered by Dr. Starzl has been modified, the basic technique remains essentially unchanged. The operation has three phases:

1. dissection to access the patient's liver
2. removal of the patient's liver
3. connecting the donated liver

First, the surgeon meticulously dissects tissues and promptly controls bleeding vessels to expose the patient's liver. This process takes about one to two hours. Blood loss ranges from zero to five pints of red blood cells.

In the next phase, the surgeon clamps the blood vessels supplying your liver and removes the liver. Then the surgeon and anesthesiologist work together to maintain adequate blood clotting factors. The anesthesiologist carefully monitors your blood and blood pressure to give you the proper fluids and blood products. In the last phase, the surgeon positions the donor liver in your abdomen and sews the blood vessels together. This procedure takes from one-and-a-half to three hours; blood loss ranges from zero to five pints.

Once all the vessels are connected, the surgeon must unclamp the main vessels. After unclamping, one of the more critical periods of the procedure begins—especially if your blood clotting is poor. After you stabilize, your surgeon connects your bile duct to the donor bile duct and removes the donor gallbladder.

Livers typically begin to function immediately after their blood supply is established. Clotting improves, and the liver makes bile on the operating table!

"The most critical moment in the operation," says University of Colorado's Chief of Transplantation, Dr. Igal Kam, "is when we release the clamps holding the vessels going to the new liver, and the new liver changes in color from pale or dark brown to a more pink-brown, because new blood is flowing to the liver. When we see the yellow-brown bile start to appear from the bile duct, we can relax because we know the liver is going to work. There's no room for mistakes in this procedure.

"About 40 to 50 percent of patients go off the respirator in the operating room and we can talk to them. After six to eight hours of surgery, it's great to talk to the patient. We deal with very sick people who sometimes have only hours to live. After the transplant, then we see the miracle."

The Hospital Stay. After the operation you may be monitored in an intensive care unit (ICU) where the staff is specifically trained to manage this early post-transplant period. Patients who are very stable may bypass the ICU and transfer from recovery room directly to the transplant inpatient floor. If you are transferred to the ICU and have no complications, you'll spend 24 to 48 hours in the ICU and then transfer to the inpatient transplant unit.

In intensive care I was in la-la land from the prednisone IV. For two days I thought I was in an alien spaceship. Other patients were in the

*ship, and that's how they were making us well. My vision was foggy.
Everything sounded as if it came from a long metal tube, echoing, dis-
torted. But I was happy, fine with that.*

*When I went to a regular room, I was still foggy and doped up. It
was uncomfortable, not painful. I was cranky, though—had some major
mood swings. After four days, they got me moving again. On my first
walk, the IV stand got away from me, and I almost fell on my face. Then
I progressed to day passes—went out for a few hours and came back. I
was there two-and-a-half weeks.*

Harry

*My legs were like tree trunks, they were so swollen with fluid. You
couldn't tell I had five toes; it looked like one big toe. A week after the
surgery, I had lost 60 pounds. The doctors would come in and tickle my
toes, just for fun.*

Janet

Usually, patients stay in the hospital from five to 20 days depending
on their condition. Some people require extensive rehabilitation, such as
physical therapy or nursing, due to their weakened situation before the
transplant.

After discharge you'll be monitored in transplant outpatient clinics
for a few weeks to a few months, and then you'll return to the care of
your referring primary care physician or gastroenterologist. The transplant center continues to guide patient management through close
cooperation with referring physicians.

Living with a New Liver

Although highly variable from patient to patient, most people require
from three to six months to physically recover from surgery and adjust
to new medications. An inspiration to transplant athletes, Chris Klug, a
28-year-old American snowboarder, took the gold in the World Cup
parallel giant slalom on January 17, 2001—less than nine months after
his liver transplant for primary sclerosing cholangitis!

Liver transplantation is a profound event that affects every part of a
patient's life—the mind as well as the body. Patients must learn to live

with lifelong medications, deal with the fear of rejection of the organ, and come to terms with a profound physical and psychological transformation.

Medications to Prevent Rejection. After the transplant, you need to take medications for the rest of your life to prevent your immune system from rejecting your new liver. The medications are called immunosuppressants and include the following: cyclosporine (Sandimmune®, Neoral®), tacrolimus (Prograf®), sirolimus (Rapamune®) azathioprine (Imuran®), steroids (Prednisone®, Solumedrol®), and mycophenolate mofetil (Cellcept®).

Most patients take either cyclosporine, tacrolimus, or sirolimus as primary therapy, and use the other agents to strengthen the anti-rejection effect. In the first six to 12 months it's common to take two or three anti-rejection medications. After that period most patients remain on cyclosporine, tacrolimus, or sirolimus, or tacrolimus either alone or in combination with low-dose Prednisone®.

> So many pills! I had eight of one kind. Taking my medication was like eating a snack. When I went to the pharmacy to pick up my first prescription, they gave it to me in a shopping bag—and then another little bag.
>
> The bill was $1,668 the first month. Ten months later, it's down to about $300.
>
> *Al*

Although the medications have side effects, most of them are dose-related and respond to either lowering the dose of the specific immunosuppressant or changing to another medication.

Never change doses by yourself. All dose adjustments of immunosuppressants require the supervision of your doctor. If you take too little immunosuppression, you run the risk of rejecting your liver transplant. If you take too much immunosuppression, you risk infection, renal (kidney) failure, hypertension, hyperlipidemia (excess blood cholesterol and fat), and diabetes mellitus.

Managing Complications. It's essential that your transplant team supervise you closely during your post-transplant outpatient care. The most concerning problems are rejection and recurrence of hepatitis C.

If rejection occurs, it typically does so within the first three months of the transplant and is detected by a rise in liver enzymes. Elevations of liver enzymes and bilirubin occur, although the first change noted is usually an increase in AST. In some cases, rejection is very mild and does not require additional immunosuppressive treatment. In more severe cases of rejection, the patient may experience fever (up to 102°F), poor appetite, fatigue, and malaise.

> *When my wife had a transplant, I was more scared than she was. I still have fear. If she gets sick, even a common cold or the flu, I still get scared. This is our second chance; there has to be a reason.*
>
> *Roger*

Nearly all rejections occur within three months of transplantation, but occasionally rejection happens later. "Late rejection" usually results from low levels of immunosuppressive therapy due to improper dosing, addition of a new medication, or development of a simultaneous illness such as diarrhea or liver dysfunction. Rejection usually responds to intravenous steroids or other strategies (OKT3).

Recurrent episodes of hepatitis C in post-transplant cases are often mistaken for rejection. Recurrent hepatitis C must be carefully considered before one embarks on a course to treat rejection.

You should expect hepatitis C to infect the liver transplant. We don't yet know how to prevent this. Pre- or post-transplant treatment with interferon- or ribavirin-based therapy is under evaluation but is often not practical because pre-transplant patients have low white blood cell counts, low platelets, and a liver that's in poor condition. In addition, no immunoglobulin preparations exist that inactivate hepatitis C.

When hepatitis C recurs, patients usually don't have symptoms and doctors detect it as an increase in blood levels of liver enzymes as early as one week after the transplant. Recurrent hepatitis C is often confused with rejection since the histologic features of rejection and hepatitis C on liver biopsies overlap considerably. Often, one must treat the patient based upon clinical impression and experience.

How do patients with hepatitis C fare after liver transplantation? Many, perhaps the majority, do extremely well with little evidence of significant damage over years of follow-up. In fact, the five-year survival after liver transplant is similar to the survival of patients transplanted for

other reasons (Figure 10A). However, some patients (less than 10 percent) have aggressive recurrence and may develop significant fibrosis or
even cirrhosis within two years. Others have an intermediate course
with various degrees of liver damage and dysfunction.

FIGURE IOA.   SURVIVAL OF PATIENTS WITH END–STAGE HCV
WHO UNDERGO LIVER TRANSPLANTATION IS
SIMILAR TO TRANSPLANTED NON–HCV PATIENTS.

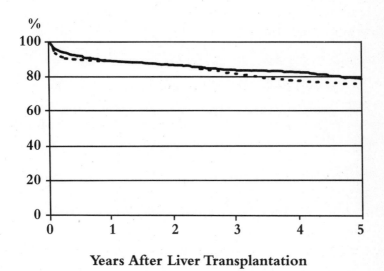

Years After Liver Transplantation

The post-transplant survival of HCV (HCV positive, N=117, solid line)
and non-HCV (HCV negative, N=317, dashed line) patients transplanted
at the University of Colorado between November 1988 and September
1998 is shown. For at least five years, there is no difference in survival
between these two groups.

Psychological Transformation. Post-transplant patients go
through a period of accepting the "gift of life." The feelings are common
to everyone and include curiosity about the donor, feelings of guilt that
someone had to die so they could live, and a sense of indebtedness—of
feeling overwhelmed and struggling with how to repay an enormous
gift.

Michael Talamantes, transplant social worker at the University of Colorado Health Sciences Center, says that patients often write a letter of thanks to the donor's family. The donor's identity is kept confidential, so the letter is sent through official channels. If the donor's family members wish to reply, they will. And if not, it's important to respect their privacy.

Feelings of guilt over the donor's death take time to work through. Although it seems obvious that the donor's death is independent of your need for a liver, the feelings are almost universal.

> *I'm small, so I got a liver from a young boy. It blew my mind. What happened to that young man that he passed away? He was only 16 years old, still a baby. It makes me feel bad because I've been through it all.*
>
> *At first I got depressed. Then I thought maybe that's why I'm doing so well—because I've got a young, healthy liver. Finally, I said, the Lord must have wanted it this way. When I get better, I'll write to his parents....*
>
> *Tomas*

The sense of indebtedness is often overwhelming. Some people do community service or visit patients in the hospital who are awaiting transplants. Every patient is touched in some way.

> *When I got the call for my liver, my heart went down to my toes. I was really scared. I went into the hospital restroom and confessed all my sins, restored my soul.*
>
> *Afterwards, when I recovered, I thought how beautiful the trees looked and how beautiful even the weeds looked. I went back to that restroom and thanked the Lord.*
>
> *Tomas*

As in every new experience, you may have contradictory feelings. It's important to pay attention to them.

Everyone talks about the "gift of life." I don't feel that way. To me, $300,000 doesn't qualify as a gift!

Sonya

It's a gift. It's unfortunate that the donor had to die, but I'm not the cause of it. Before I knew I would need a transplant, I put on my license I was a donor. I made the same decision, and I honor my donor's decision.

Sandy

Whatever normal, contradictory feelings you have, you need to sort through them to adjust to your new sense of yourself. To complicate matters, you may get mixed messages from others. Are you a hero, a biotechnological miracle, or does your boss see you as damaged goods, a drain on the company's health insurance? Whatever your experiences, they are profound indeed. You are not alone in wrestling with these issues.

People who haven't had a transplant don't understand. All they see is machinery and medicines. It's really important to talk. If someone calls me, it cheers me up to just listen, to say I was there. It can't get any better than that—to talk to someone who's been there, done that.

Evie

Improved Survival Rates

The heartening news is that survival rates have increased due to advances in immunosuppression (beginning with cyclosporine in 1979) and the team approach to liver transplantation. Before cyclosporine, patients were treated with high doses of Prednisone and azathioprine. Procedures, such as thoracic duct drainage, splenectomy, and anti-lymphocyte immunoglobulin injections, were used to further suppress the immune system and prevent rejection. Before 1979, results were poor: 32 percent of patients survived one year and only 22 percent survived 30 months.

The picture has changed dramatically. Liver transplant results show that average one- and three-year patient survival rates in the U.S. from 1988 to 1995 were 77 and 68 percent respectively. During the same period the average one- and three-year survival rates in Europe were 73 and 65 percent. Our results at the University of Colorado compared favorably to the overall results in both the U.S. and Europe: one- and three-year patient survival rates were 86 and 78 percent. Survival of hepatitis C patients is similar to non-hepatitis C patients undergoing liver transplantation (see Figure 10A).

The reality is, however, that not all patients survive. Deaths occurring within the first six months are due to nonfunction of the donor's liver, clotting of the main artery to the liver, infection, multi-organ failure, or rejection. When deaths occur later after the transplant, they are more commonly due to malignancy or complications of atherosclerosis and rarely to rejection or infection.

The outlook is very hopeful. We anticipate that current immunosuppressive protocols will reduce adverse metabolic effects and continue to improve the long-term outlook for transplant recipients. (Since 1995 one-year survival rates at the University of Colorado exceed 90 percent.) Our ultimate goal, of course, is to restore you to your normal life.

How Organs Are Allocated

UNOS. In the United States, the United Network for Organ-Sharing (UNOS) regulates the distribution or allocation of donor organs. Here's how it works.

The United States is divided into 11 regions for organ procurement and allocation. Several local organ procurement organizations (OPOs) exist within each region. When a patient is approved for transplantation, he or she is placed on local, regional, and national waiting lists. Typically, more than 80 percent of recipients receive organs from local donors.

Listing Status. A patient placed on the waiting list is given a UNOS status, or priority, based upon severity of disease. UNOS 1 is the most urgent status. Patients in this category have acute irreversible liver failure and are not likely to survive beyond seven days without transplantation. Patients at UNOS 2a are given the next priority. These patients have chronic liver disease but are hospitalized in the intensive care unit with projected survival of less than 14 days. UNOS 2b patients are more stable but with signs of liver decompensation (see Chapter 4). Patients listed at UNOS 3 are typically stable at home and not likely to undergo transplantation.

As of this writing, UNOS is evaluating the Mayo End-Stage Liver Disease score (MELD) for allocating organs. MELD score is calcualted for each patient based upon diagnosis and blood tests. Priority for transplant will be given to patients wtih the highest MELD score.

As the waiting list continues to expand, will a shortage of donors lead to increasing numbers of people dying while they wait for a liver? The number of patients listed more than quintupled from 1988 to 1998, but the number of liver transplants only doubled. In 1988, 214 patients on the waiting list died. In 1994, 694 patients died, and in 2000, 1,636 died. As a society we need to find solutions to the organ shortage.

Centers of Excellence. UNOS displays the results for liver transplantation in the United States on its continually updated website, www.unos.org. Patient and graft survivals for one- and three-year outcomes are given in combined totals and for each individual center. Results are also adjusted for differences in patient populations according to variables known to influence outcome after liver transplantation: UNOS listing status, diagnosis of fulminant hepatic failure, age, renal failure, presence of hepatitis B, and presence of primary liver cancer. Using this stratification method, results from each center can be compared to the expected outcome. Intuitively, one could suggest that this analysis identifies true "centers of excellence," because it is based solely upon adjusted medical outcomes.

Medicare was the first to put into practice the concept of centers of excellence in liver transplantation. Additional third-party insurers, such as Blue Cross/Blue Shield, Prudential, United Resource Network, and Kaiser Permanente use similar criteria. With the explosion of HMOs the criteria for designating centers of excellence are more a mixture of medical outcome and economic impact. Adoption of standardized medical criteria for designation of "centers of excellence" would eliminate the potential that a given program could be an insurer's transplant center by simply offering the lowest price.

Many people have suggested that the current number of 117 transplant programs is far in excess of what the donor organ pool can provide. More than half the programs in the U.S. perform fewer than 20 liver transplants per year; 75 percent of all liver transplants are performed by only 25 percent of the programs.

A recent publication by UNOS in *The New England Journal of Medicine* confirms that transplant teams that perform more than 20 transplants per year achieve optimal patient and graft survival. According to this analysis, the chance to die after liver transplantation is almost twice as great when the transplant is done by a program performing fewer than 20 transplants per year. Because more than half the programs in the U.S. perform fewer than 20 transplants a year, one must question the wisdom of encouraging the proliferation of transplant centers.

Some states have invoked the concept of "certification of need" to ensure a balance between the regional need for transplantation and the number of transplant centers. Further increases in the number of transplant centers should be discouraged unless dictated by regional need.

Resource: Call the toll-free UNOS patient information number at 1-888-TXINFO1 (1-888-894-6361); website: www.unos.org. To request free single copies of the following brochures, write to UNOS, P.O. Box 13770, Richmond, VA 23286-2659: *What Every Patient Needs to Know; Information for Patients; Share Your Life. Share Your Decision*^{sm}*; Vital Connections.*

Resource: Updated Waitlist and Transplant Summary Reports, statistics by state, region, or individual hospitals, and other information are available on the UNOS website: www.unos.org. To order free printed versions of the *1997 Report of Center Specific Graft and Patient Survival Rates* by individual volume or complete seven-volume set (there is a shipping charge), contact the UNOS Professional Services Department at 804-330-8541.

Resource: Regional organ recovery organizations are a good source of information. To locate your region's organization, call the UNOS patient information number listed above.

Resource: For information on national organizations and local coalitions that educate the public about organ donation, call the Coalition on Donation: 804-330-8620; email: coalition@unos.org; website: www.shareyourlife.org. You may also request a free brochure on organ donation from the Coalition by calling 1-800-355-SHARE.

Resource: For a free *Transplant Support Group Directory* (of more than 300 pre- and post-transplant support groups nationwide) and a sample copy of the *Solstice* newsletter (dedicated to organ transplantation), call Chronimed Pharmacy: 1-800-888-5753 and ask for a patient specialist.

Resource: For free pamphlets and information about transplants and organ donation, call a nationwide support group for transplant patients and their families, Transplant Recipients International Organization (TRIO): 1-800-TRIO-386.

Resource: A uniform donor card is enclosed in this book. Discuss organ and tissue donation with family members. After completing and signing the Uniform Donor Card, be sure to have your signature witnessed by two people.

To every thing there is a season, and a time to every purpose under the heaven...

A time to weep, and a time to laugh; a time to mourn, and a time to dance...

Ecclesiastes

11

LIVER CANCER
Are You At Risk?

Just the word "cancer" scares me. I thought I'd die. I have four kids, and I was just terrified.

Six years after I was diagnosed with hepatitis C, I weighed 89 pounds. I had no appetite. My liver enzymes went sky high. The doctors sent me for a CT scan and found liver cancer. Thank God they put me on the transplant waiting list because it gave me hope.

After ten months I got my new liver. My weight's back; I'm 120 pounds. The cancer blood tests are good. "How's the hepatitis C?" I ask my nurse. "Very quiet," she says.

See this bulge here? My new liver is too large for me. But I just wear big shirts—and I'm still alive!

Carolyn

MOST OF MY PATIENTS DON'T realize that hepatitis C can cause liver cancer (hepatoma). But before you panic or worry unnecessarily, consider the following:

1. Only a minority of patients with hepatitis C will ever develop liver cancer.
2. Effective therapies exist for tumors detected early.

3. Liver cancer is almost entirely restricted to those with advanced liver disease who have extensive fibrosis (stage III) or cirrhosis.

Of course, you're wondering if *you* are in danger. This chapter provides you with information regarding risk factors, warning signs, screening and diagnostic tests for liver cancer, and results of current treatment. Here are the topics I'll cover:

- Overview: What Is Liver Cancer?
    Primary Liver Cancer (Hepatoma)
    Secondary Liver Cancer
    Is Primary Liver Cancer on the Rise?
- Common Risk Factors
    Stage of Hepatitis C
    Duration of Infection
    Other Liver Diseases
    Viral Genotype, Viral RNA Level, Quasispecies
- Interferon: Does It Reduce the Risk of Primary Liver Cancer?
- Warning Signs
    No Symptoms but with Underlying Cirrhosis
    Deterioration in Liver Function
    Pain
    Sudden Development of Portal Hypertension
    Other Symptoms
- Testing
    Early Screening Guidelines
        Blood Tests (Serial Measurement of Alpha-fetoprotein)
        Radiologic Imaging
    Diagnostic Tests
- Treatment
    Cancer Staging
        Early Stage
        Advanced Stage
        Metastic Liver Cancer
    Hepatic Resection
    Transplantation
    Chemoembolization
    High-Frequency Radio Waves (Radiofrequency Tumor Ablation)
    Alcohol Injection, Cryosurgery
    Chemotherapy

• Summary

Overview: What Is Liver Cancer?

Primary Liver Cancer (Hepatoma). Primary liver cancer, also known as hepatoma or hepatocellular carcinoma, is a malignant tumor that originates within the liver. Nearly all hepatomas originate from cells composed of the main tissue of the liver (hepatocytes), rather than from cells of the biliary tract, fibrous tissue, blood vessels, or fat.

Secondary Liver Cancer. In the United States, primary liver cancer is relatively rare. Most cancers migrate to the liver, are called secondary cancers, and have their primary site in other organs of the body, such as the colon, breast, or lung. Secondary liver cancers frequently appear as multiple liver masses, while primary liver cancers commonly appear as a solitary mass.

Physicians distinguish secondary from primary liver cancers by imaging the liver (ultrasonography, CT, MRT) and biopsing the tissue. The finding of secondary liver cancer means that tumor cells have traveled far from their primary site, typically indicating a poor chance of survival. Liver transplantation is not indicated for secondary liver cancers.

Is Primary Liver Cancer on the Rise? In the past, primary liver cancers were so rare that doctors often selected these cases for presentation at medical Grand Rounds lectures. Today, we diagnose primary liver cancer with increasing frequency, especially in patients with chronic hepatitis C. The Centers for Disease Control and Prevention report that the incidence of hepatoma increased from 1.4 to 2.4 per 100,000 people between 1979 and 1995.

In my own state of Colorado, the number of cases of hepatoma doubled from 1988 to 1998. The number of patients with hepatoma presented to the Tumor Board at University Hospital was six in 1988 and 24 in 1997. Existing data suggest that the increase in primary liver cancer is directly related to chronic hepatitis C.

Common Risk Factors

Stage of Hepatitis C. The most important predictor of liver cancer is the condition of the liver tissue (histologic stage). Noncirrhotic patients have a low risk, patients with extensive fibrosis (stage III) run an intermediate risk, and those with cirrhosis are at greatest risk.

Five studies have examined the risk of developing liver cancer in patients with established cirrhosis due to hepatitis C. The annual incidence of hepatoma ranged from 1.2 percent per year to 9.5 percent per year. Patients with early cirrhosis probably have a risk of 1 percent per year, and those with advanced cirrhosis have a risk closer to 5 to 10 percent per year.

I believe that noncirrhotic patients without significant fibrosis are at low risk for this complication and do not have to undergo screening for liver tumors. In contrast, patients with cirrhosis run a considerable lifetime risk of developing hepatoma and should undergo screening. Cirrhotic patients who develop sudden onset of decompensation (see Chapter 4), should undergo diagnostic studies to rule out liver cancer.

Duration of Infection. Most data suggest that the median time period for developing hepatoma is approximately 30 years from the date of infection and 10 years after the onset of cirrhosis. If you don't have cirrhosis but have had hepatitis C for 30 years, you may still be at risk for liver cancer. However, this issue has not been adequately studied and the exact risk is unknown.

Other Liver Diseases. Any liver disease that hastens the development of cirrhosis may also increase the likelihood of developing hepatoma. The three most common concurrent hepatic diseases in hepatitis C patients that accelerate disease progression are chronic alcohol use, hepatitis B, and genetic hemochromatosis.

Multiple studies have now conclusively demonstrated that patients with hepatitis C who drink alcohol add fuel to the hepatitis C fire. Chronic daily consumption of alcohol is associated with acceleration to cirrhosis, increased risk for liver failure, increased risk for needing liver transplantation, and increased risk for development of liver cancer. Similar risks have been observed in patients with hepatitis C who are co-infected with hepatitis B. In addition, hemochromatosis, the most common genetic liver disease, causes excessive accumulation of iron in the liver, which also accelerates liver disease due to hepatitis C and, therefore, potentially increases the risk of liver cancer.

Viral Genotype, Viral RNA Level, Quasispecies. Genotype 1b has been associated with longer duration of disease, more aggressive disease activity, increased likelihood for progression to cirrhosis, and increased need for liver transplantation. Therefore, it's not surprising that this genotype has also been linked to hepatoma, though it is not known whether genotype 1b is an independent predictor of liver cancer. Levels of HCV-RNA in the blood and the diversity of the hepatitis C virus RNAs (quasispecies) have not been proven to correlate with the risk of developing hepatoma.

Interferon: Does It Reduce the Risk of Primary Liver Cancer?

Interferon treatment may reduce the risk of hepatoma, even when treatment does not normalize the liver enzymes or eradicate the hepatitis C virus. Five uncontrolled studies suggested the following:

1. Sustained response to interferon (normal ALT and negative HCV-RNA) may eliminate the risk of hepatoma.
2. Nonresponders to interferon (abnormal ALT and positive HCV-RNA) may have a lower risk of hepatoma than patients who were never treated—3 to 5 percent versus 10 to 38 percent.

WARNING: The above studies were uncontrolled and retrospective. Bias in reporting or treating patients may have yielded the false impression of a positive effect of interferon when, in fact, the treatment may have been ineffective. Randomized, controlled, prospective trials, such as the Hepatitis C Antiviral Long-Term Treatment Against Cirrhosis (HALT C), are needed to answer the question of whether interferon therapy effectively prevents hepatoma in patients with chronic hepatitis C.

The HALT C study, sponsored by the National Institute of Diabetes & Digestive & Kidney Diseases, National Institutes of Health, Bethesda, MD, was designed to answer the question of whether maintenance interferon therapy could slow down progression or reduce the risk of liver cancer. Ten U.S. sites are participating.

Resource: For additional information about HALT C, contact the NIH clinical center's patient recruitment and public liason office at 1-800-411-1222 (TTY: 1-866-411-1010). NIH website: www.nih.gov

Warning Signs

No Symptoms but with Underlying Cirrhosis. Many patients develop hepatoma without any changes in symptoms or obvious progression of their disease. That's why I recommend screening tests, such as alpha-fetoprotein and ultrasonography for all patients with bridging fibrosis (stage III) or cirrhosis. Detection of hepatoma with screening tests may result in more effective treatment and better outcomes.

Deterioration in Liver Function. A stable cirrhotic patient may be fully employed, have normal levels of energy, conduct normal social activities, and have stable liver tests. When such a patient develops hepatoma, liver function may deteriorate for no other apparent reason. Signs of deterioration are increasing fatigue, mental confusion (encephalopathy), fluid retention (ascites, edema), or gastrointestinal bleeding. Alternatively, the patient's liver tests may suddenly deteriorate with rising bilirubin, diminishing clotting factors, increase in liver enzymes, and drop in serum albumin. Some patients experience only a loss of appetite, fever, and unexplained weight loss.

> *In March my husband was starting to feel tired. A checkup showed his blood work was fine, and the liver scan came back great.*
>
> *In mid-April he ran twice around the track and was exhausted. He said he hurt his back and took muscle relaxers. A week later, he vomited blood all over the bathroom floor. He told me it was just juice mixed with the medicine—but I saw blood clots.*
>
> *At the hospital they found out his stomach was bleeding. A CT scan showed liver cancer. Since his first test, the thing had grown to over 20 centimeters. They couldn't operate on the cancer because it was the size of his liver.*
>
> *"No go," said the doctor. "It's too big."*
>
> *Claudine*

Pain. A tumor can grow rapidly, causing the liver capsule to expand, and tumor cells can invade adjacent nerve roots, blood vessels, and lymphatics. As the hepatoma enlarges and impinges on adjacent structures, it can create significant pain and discomfort. Development of persistent moderate to severe pain in the right upper quadrant of the abdomen in a patient with cirrhosis may point to the diagnosis of hepatoma.

Sudden Development of Portal Hypertension. Hepatoma is a vascular tumor and often invades vascular structures, such as blood or fluid-bearing vessels or ducts. If the tumor enters the portal vein, it may plug the vessel or cause blood clotting that blocks the vein. An acute rise in portal pressure related to this blockage may result in an upper gastrointestinal bleed (variceal hemorrhage), swelling of the abdomen (ascites) or ankles, worsening of existing ascites, development of diuretic-resistant ascites, mental confusion (encephalopathy), or worsening of existing encephalopathy.

> *My husband's final request was to see the ocean one more time. He wanted to say goodbye to his sisters in California. The night before our flight, I heard him yell. Vomiting blood, he collapsed at the bottom of the stairs.*
>
> *At the hospital I freaked out, and I was crying, crying. The pain was like a monster in his stomach. "No, no," he said, "I want to go see my sisters!" That whole last week he talked about God. He knew he'd be with the Lord when he died.*
>
> *His sisters flew in. He was still awake and able to recognize them. The next morning he got very confused. He died that night.*
>
> *Annie*

Other Symptoms. Patients may attribute certain nonspecific symptoms (fatigue, loss of appetite, poor energy) to their ongoing hepatitis C when the symptoms may be related to emergence of hepatoma. These patients often delay notifying their physicians for several months. Such a delay may convert a potentially treatable tumor to one that has spread beyond the confines of the liver and may no longer be treatable.

Testing

Early Screening Guidelines. Doctors have not yet established guidelines for screening for hepatoma in patients with hepatitis C. However, recent clinical trials have indicated that screening with both alpha-fetoprotein and ultrasonography detects early tumors and results in improved patient survival. Nonetheless, many of my comments on screening come from my own experience and represent my bias regarding the most cost-effective and sensitive approach to this problem.

Again, I want to emphasize that most patients with hepatitis C will not develop primary liver cancer. Noncirrhotic patients appear to be at an exceedingly low risk, and only those with advanced fibrosis or cirrhosis who have had the disease for more than 20 years are at excess risk. Therefore, all comments regarding screening apply only to patients with bridging fibrosis (stage III) or cirrhosis.

The two screening tests doctors use to detect liver cancer are (1) blood tests (serial measurement of alpha-fetoprotein) and (2) radiologic imaging.

1. **Blood Tests (Serial Measurement of Alpha-fetoprotein).** Hepatoma cells synthesize a protein called alpha-fetoprotein and release the protein into the bloodstream. A very high alpha-fetoprotein [>500 nanograms (ng) per milliliter (ml)] or a sustained rise in alpha-fetoprotein on serial measurements (with the last value > 150 ng/ml) may predict the development of hepatoma. A subtype of alpha-fetoprotein (L3) may be more specific for cancer. Other blood tests, such as PIVKA-II, are under investigation.

   The accuracy of alpha-fetoprotein, used alone, in predicting hepatoma is poor. Therefore, doctors may order supplemental radiologic tests, biopsies, or even a surgical incision (laparotomy). In addition, 20 to 50 percent of the hepatomas that occur in patients with hepatitis C may lack the ability to produce alpha-fetoprotein. In such cases, the tumors progress undetected by the serial alpha-fetoprotein measurements. Radiologic imaging of the liver is required to screen for these tumors.

2. **Radiologic Imaging.** Although CT scans and magnetic resonance imaging (MRI) with enhancing agents may be slightly more sensitive than ultrasonography, they are prohibitively expensive for use in screening. Ultrasonography, on the other hand, which can detect the majority of early hepatomas, is much less costly and is the radiologic screening choice.

   I currently advise my cirrhotic patients and those with extensive fibrosis to have alpha-fetoprotein measurements and ultrasonography of the liver every six months.

   Diagnostic Tests. If screening tests detect a lesion that might be cancerous, doctors may biopsy the mass with the guidance of ultrasonography or CT. Other imaging studies (CT, MRI, or angiography) can detect early hepatoma in the patient with rising alpha-fetoprotein or worsening of symptoms when ultrasonography fails to reveal a definite lesion. The type of imaging study is ordered at your physician's discretion.

Treatment

Cancer Staging. In order to select proper treatment, the physician must determine the stage of the hepatoma. This is usually done with radiologic imaging, laparoscopy, or abdominal exploratory surgery.

1. **Early Stage.** Patients with a solitary tumor less than five centimeters in diameter or patients with up to three tumors, all less than three centimeters in diameter, may be candidates for surgery to remove the tumor (hepatic resection) or liver transplantation. Recurrence of the tumor is common if resection is performed. Cure and excellent long-term survival are the rule with liver transplantation.

2. **Advanced Stage.** More advanced stages of hepatoma usually represent multiple tumor nodules involving one or both liver lobes. The tumor may have invaded the main liver vessels. Advanced stage tumors have a poorer prognosis, and typically doctors do not advise resection or transplantation.

   Most patients cannot undergo resection due to the extensive nature of the disease and the risk of precipitating liver failure because of underlying cirrhosis. Only a small subgroup is considered for transplantation. However, the outcome after liver transplantation is poor for patients with advanced stage hepatomas, because of recurrence of cancer. Patients with advanced stage cancer are considered for palliative treatment with either chemoembolization, cryosurgery, or radiofrequency thermal ablation.

3. **Metastatic Liver Cancer.** Patients with widespread tumor that has metastasized (spread) beyond the confines of the liver are not candidates for surgery, transplantation, cryotherapy, or chemoembolization. They are evaluated only for standard chemotherapy.

Hepatic Resection. Surgeons achieve the best results in the treatment of hepatoma when they perform a liver resection to surgically remove a solitary tumor (less than five centimeters) in a patient with a noncirrhotic liver. These patients may be cured of their cancer and usually enjoy long-term survival.

However, this represents an uncommon clinical scenario when it comes to hepatoma in patients with hepatitis C. As I have already mentioned, the patient with hepatitis C who develops a liver cancer usually has cirrhosis and a disease duration of hepatitis C for greater than 30 years.

My wife was prepped for surgery. First, the doctors did a biopsy. "The other side of her liver is all cirrhosed," they told me. "You have 30 days before she gets real sick." They said to wind up her affairs—wills and such—and see to our family.

When we got home, she only had energy to go to the post office and the bank. And that was it for the day.

Owen

Unfortunately, cirrhosis precludes a successful resection because resections for hepatoma usually require removing 25 to 75 percent of the liver tissue. A normal liver can tolerate a massive resection since regeneration is rapid (usually within 12 weeks) and the remaining liver cells are functioning normally. That's not the case when a person has cirrhosis and hepatitis C. The remaining liver cannot effectively regenerate, and its function is severely impaired. When a surgeon performs a large resection on a cirrhotic patient, the operation may lead to liver failure. For these reasons liver resections are usually restricted to patients without cirrhosis or to those cirrhotic patients who have no evidence of clinical or biochemical deterioration in liver function or portal hypertension.

Transplantation. Results from a number of centers agree: Cirrhotic patients with solitary liver cancers, small in size (less than five centimeters in diameter) or up to three tumors (all less than three centimeters in diameter), should be considered for transplantation.

Successful transplantation may also be performed on patients with multiple tumor nodules (all less than two centimeters) that are restricted to one hepatic lobe with no evidence of invasion of blood vessels. Although these two groups of patients can expect long-term, tumor-free survival, those with advanced stages of hepatoma or metastatic disease almost uniformly experience early post-transplant recurrence of tumor and death from metastatic disease. Transplantation is not indicated for the latter patients.

Even for hepatomas in favorable stages, time can run out. Most of the data that deals with successful transplants for hepatoma come from an era of relatively greater availability of donor livers. That situation no longer exists in this country. The U.S. waiting list for liver transplantation continues to expand. As of July 2001, 18,028 people were on the list, but only about 4,500 liver transplants are performed annually.

Patients with hepatoma are at a distinct disadvantage as they wait for a liver. The tumor will grow with time, spread to adjacent areas of the liver, invade blood vessels, and prevent the patient from continuing as a transplant candidate. Patients with hepatoma are currently given higher UNOS status (2b) but also need to be considered for living-donor liver transplantation (see Chapter 9).

Given current statistics, I project that by the year 2015 the U.S. waiting list will contain 30,000 to 45,000 patients. The majority of these patients will have hepatitis C, and a sizeable number will develop hepatoma while waiting for a donor liver.

> Four years ago, the doctor thought my liver was bruised from all the biopsies I had. He said it could be a hepatoma, but I didn't know that meant cancer. When the doctor told me the biopsy was positive, all the blood ran out of my face; my knees gave out. Three months later, I got my liver transplant.
>
> I remember hallucinating about dying when I was in the hospital. I saw the place where I go fishing—a nice, peaceful place with green grass and a stream running through. I wanted to lie down, go to sleep, give up.
>
> But I had just rebuilt my Harley-Davidson®. In my fantasy I got on my cycle and rode it for two days down this highway with a white dotted line in the middle of the road. I heard the roar of the exhaust and smelled the pine trees.
>
> It was the turning point. I didn't quit fighting—and the cancer is gone. That dang Harley-Davidson® saved my life. I feel like I won the lotto!
>
> Jack

Chemoembolization. This procedure does not cure cancer. However, it can help destroy local tumors, reduce the tumor mass, provide significant relief, or in the case of a solitary tumor, keep the tumor from spreading outside the liver until a donor liver becomes available.

My family was 100 percent for the transplant, but my husband got so worried and scared for me, he lost 30 pounds. He was nothing but skin and bones.

They put me in the hospital and gave me chemoembolization twice. I lost all my hair. It was scary, but I made it to my transplant. I have a lot of faith in God. That's what got me through—that and my family.

Krista

The technique involves placing a catheter through a vessel in the groin (the femoral artery) and advancing it into the liver's main artery (the hepatic artery). Then a special form of chemotherapy is infused through the catheter into the artery feeding the tumor. Both normal and hepatoma cells take up the chemotherapy, but cancer cells do not excrete it. Because cancer cells retain the chemotherapy for a prolonged time, they are destroyed.

In the absence of resection or transplantation, chemoembolization is not curative, and the patient should understand that the tumor will probably recur. Nonetheless, chemoembolization of the tumor has been associated with prolonged survival and reduced symptoms of pain and weight loss. In transplant candidates, chemoembolization may sustain the patient until successful transplantation can take place.

High-Frequency Radio Waves (Radiofrequency Tumor Ablation). This treatment of hepatoma remains under study. The technique involves CT-guided puncture of the hepatoma and positioning the prongs of a special instrument within the tumor mass. High-frequency radio waves (near the microwave limit) generated within the tumor mass destroy the tumor. Overall effectiveness and clinical outcome of this treatment for hepatoma remain to be defined.

Alcohol Injection, Cryosurgery. These two approaches are also limited to hepatomas that cannot be resected or transplanted. The goal of these treatments is to reduce tumor size and relieve painful symptoms.

Alcohol injection is done with the guidance of a CT scan to ensure proper placement of the treatment catheter within the tumor. Absolute alcohol dehydrates the tissues, causing the immediate death of cells, and starts a clotting process within the tumor that destroys it.

Cryosurgery involves the use of a flexible fiberoptic instrument (laparoscopy) with the guidance of an ultrasound probe to properly position the cryosurgical instrument within the tumor. When the probe is positioned, the tumor cells are destroyed by freezing.

Chemotherapy. Hepatoma is one of the most resistant tumors to both radiation and chemotherapy. Early experience with external beam radiation suggested that doses of radiation required for effective anti-tumor activity exceeded safety standards. In addition, clinical experience with radiation therapy of hepatomas was uniformly dismal and disappointing. For this reason, radiation is employed only rarely in the treatment of these tumors. Some evidence suggests that chemotherapy can be partially effective in reducing tumor burden and relieving symptoms.

Summary

Primary liver cancer is an extremely serious, life-threatening complication of chronic hepatitis C, but it occurs mainly in patients with advanced disease and cirrhosis. Hepatitis C patients with bridging fibrosis or cirrhosis should be aware of the danger of liver cancer, undergo screening by their physician, and know the warning signs.

Early hepatoma is treatable, but most patients with large tumors or multiple tumors cannot be treated by liver resection or transplantation. Cirrhotic patients with solitary and small hepatomas should be considered for early liver transplantation and possibly living-donor transplantation. A number of new approaches can reduce but not cure inoperable tumors: chemoembolization, radiofrequency thermal ablation, alcohol ablation, cryosurgery, and systemic chemotherapy.

Liver cancer is an increasingly important issue for hepatitis C patients, families, physicians, surgeons, transplant programs, and the health care system in general. We in the medical community know that we sorely need new ideas and new treatments.

The first wealth is health.

Emerson

1 2

CO-INFECTION WITH HIV/AIDS OR HEPATITIS B

Triple Trouble

In 1996 the doctors took me off AZT and put me on triple combination drug therapy. My T-cells went up, and my viral load went down. The nurse said they could probably keep me alive for a long time if I stayed off drugs and cocaine.

Meanwhile, two friends with AIDS killed themselves. The loneliness, deaths, and suicides were too much. Then I found out I had hepatitis C in August. I was tired all the time, so they tested me—and the tests came back reactive for hepatitis B and C.

I cried. I started reading about hepatitis C, and none of it looked good. Another virus. Now I have three viruses in my body.

Jay

THIS CHAPTER DISCUSSES two types of viral co-infections: HIV and hepatitis B. If you are battling hepatitis C, it can be devastating to discover that you have another viral infection—HIV/AIDS or hepatitis B. It is even possible that you are co-infected with three viruses simultaneously.

You know from personal experience what it means to live with one dangerous virus, and now you have to face co-infection. Nothing can prepare you for the shock. Once again, you go through the cycle of fear, anger, and denial.

Until a few years ago, doctors did not focus on treating hepatitis C in patients with AIDS because patients with AIDS had limited years to live. Also, interferon treatment affected the immune system, which was already impaired by AIDS. Now, however, the introduction of new highly active AIDS drugs (HAART therapy) has produced a growing number of HIV-infected patients with strengthened immune systems who are enjoying longer life spans. With this hopeful and encouraging development, treatment of hepatitis C in patients with HIV infection becomes a greater concern. Recently, the U.S. Public Health Service declared hepatitis an "official" opportunistic infection in patients with HIV.

Co-infection with hepatitis B alters your prognosis and raises treatment issues. Patients co-infected with hepatitis B tend to have more aggressive liver disease with a greater likelihood of progression to cirrhosis and the need for a liver transplant. Also, the risk of cancer increases. When dealing with hepatitis B and C co-infection, the doctor must assess and determine the dominant agent and tailor treatment to the dominant virus.

In this chapter, I will discuss the following topics:

- Overview of HIV Co-Infection
  What Is HIV/AIDS?
  Are You at Risk for Co-Infection?
  Testing Problems
  Population Trends
- Current Treatment of HIV Infection
  Highly Active Anti-Retroviral Therapies (HAART)
- Complications of HAART Therapy
  Effect of Hepatitis C Infection on HIV
  Effect of HIV Infection on Hepatitis C

- Does HIV Co-Infection Affect the Rate of Progression of Liver Disease?
- Antiviral Therapy of Hepatitis C in Patients Co-Infected with HIV
    Are New Treatments on the Horizon for Co-Infected Patients?
- Co-Infection with Hepatitis B
- Liver Transplantation
    Transplantation before HAART
    Transplantation after HAART
- Summary

Overview of HIV Co-Infection

What Is HIV/AIDS? The human immunodeficiency virus (HIV) destroys the immune system that helps the body fight illness and infection. HIV infects lymphocytes, the main immune cells in the body, and causes acquired immunodeficiency syndrome (AIDS). Severe damage to the immune system results in susceptibility to a wide array of infections and malignancy (cancer).

According to the Centers for Disease Control and Prevention (CDC) June 2000 figures, an estimated 800,000 to 900,000 people are living with HIV/AIDS in the United States—about 0.3 percent of the population. Worldwide, the estimated number of people living with HIV/AIDS is 36.1 million.

Are You at Risk for Co-Infection? Many people with AIDS are also infected with the hepatitis C virus (HCV) because some behaviors that transmit AIDS also transmit hepatitis C (such as sharing intravenous drug needles or receiving blood transfusions, organ transplants, or hemophilia treatment before tests screened the nation's blood supply). When AIDS patients are infected with both HIV and HCV, it is called an HIV/HCV co-infection.

In my experience, HIV treatment clinics diagnose most cases of hepatitis C and HIV co-infection because symptoms relating to HIV usually show up before those of hepatitis C. In fact, I have diagnosed unsuspected HIV in only a handful of patients with chronic hepatitis C (despite routine HIV testing of our hepatitis C population) during my years directing our hepatology clinics.

I'm a vet. In 1996 I had outpatient treatment, and my blood came back positive for HIV. The diagnosis threw me. I just gave up.

It was an avalanche. Where am I going? What am I going to do? Then this year rolled around. My doctor wanted me to take a hepatitis B shot. That's when I found out I had hepatitis C.

Joel

How many people with HIV are also infected with hepatitis C? The answer to this question is more complicated than it seems because nearly all prevalence data have relied on the results from antibody testing—not on HCV-RNA assays of viral load (see Chapter 2 for a discussion of these different types of tests).

Testing Problems. Researchers have documented that antibody tests for hepatitis C in patients with HIV may fluctuate; spontaneous conversion of hepatitis C from positive to negative antibodies may occur.

In addition, antibody tests may yield both false positive and false negative results. For example, an HIV patient may test negative to the HCV antibody but harbor the hepatitis C virus in the blood. Or, conversely, a patient could test positive to the HCV antibody but lack viral infection. False positive rates with first generation tests in this population have been reported to be as high as 50 percent. For these reasons, I recommend that all HIV patients who test positive for HCV antibody undergo confirmation of hepatitis C infection by assay of HCV-RNA. Despite these shortcomings and caveats, the data from the studies described below are still useful in identifying trends.

Population Trends. Two prospective studies examined the occurrence of the hepatitis C antibody in the blood of patients newly diagnosed with HIV. One, from the University of Toronto, found an 8 percent occurrence in a group of 224 patients. The other, from the University of California at Davis, reported an occurrence of 7 percent.

Risk of co-infection with hepatitis C relates to how HIV was acquired. Patients who acquired HIV from blood-borne routes, as opposed to sexual routes, are more likely to be co-infected with hepatitis C. Patients who acquired HIV from intravenous drug use have a greater than 50 percent chance of also harboring hepatitis C. Hemophiliacs who acquired HIV from transfusion with unpasteurized plasma-derived factor VIII concentrates have rates of co-infection of hepatitis C greater than 70 percent. These co-infection statistics are strikingly elevated when one compares them to the hepatitis C prevalence of less than 5 percent among male homosexuals with HIV who don't have a history of either transfusions or intravenous drug use.

> *When they told me I had HIV and they could keep me alive for five years tops, I was terrified. I thought I'd be dead very soon. I fell off the wagon after six months of sobriety. Figuring it didn't make any difference, I drank, I did drugs—anything to numb myself.*
> *I suppose that's how I got hepatitis C in the first place.*
>
> *Carl*

Resource: For information on co-infection with HIV and hepatitis, access this website: www.hivandhepatitis.com.

Current Treatment of HIV Infection

HIV is an RNA virus acquired by blood-borne routes or sexual activity. The virus, first identified in 1983 as the cause of AIDS, was given the name human T-cell lymphotropic virus type III (HTLV-III) in the United States because of its known association with lymphocytes. HIV infects the body's immune cells (lymphocytes), which then become dysfunctional, nonfunctional, or die, thus severely impairing the body's immune system. Before current effective anti-HIV therapy, most patients succumbed to either the ravages of infectious disease or malignancy.

> *I've known 35 people who died from AIDS since 1985. When they put me on AZT, I figured I had two years left. That's what I had seen. The only thing that kept me going was taking care of my friend Jonathon, who went blind a month before he died. It was very hard.*
>
> *Bill*

Highly Active Anti-Retroviral Therapies (HAART). Two classes of drugs, reverse transcriptase inhibitors and protease inhibitors, dramatically altered the course of HIV infection. Today, most patients with HIV are treated with a combination of three to four drugs, and they experience significant improvement.

Seven years after my HIV diagnosis, the nurses called me at work. My T-cells were 160. I had AIDS! Confused, depressed, I flunked the memory tests and a CT scan showed I had a shrinkage of the brain. They put me on AZT.

Four years later, I went on HAART. My T-cells went up. Now I'm more scared of hepatitis C than HIV. After 14 years of being HIV-positive, you learn to deal with it, but this hepatitis thing is new. I'm dealing with all that uncertainty all over again.

John

How effective are these highly active anti-retroviral therapies (HAART)? Steven C. Johnson, M.D., Associate Professor of Medicine and Director of the University Hospital HIV/AIDS Clinical Program, University of Colorado Health Sciences Center, recently reviewed outcomes over a three-year period.[1] From 1995 through 1997 the percentage of AIDS patients treated with HAART increased from less than 10 percent to over 80 percent. The rate of hospitalization fell from 6.4 to 1.1 inpatient days per patient-year. Decreases in days of hospitalization resulted in significant cost reductions. The incidence of the three major opportunistic infections (infections that develop only because of the patient's immune deficiency)—pneumocystis pneumonia, mycobacterium avium complex disease, and cytomegalovirus retinitis (CMV)—decreased dramatically. Death from opportunistic infection or advanced HIV declined markedly from 15 percent of the clinic population in 1994 to 2 percent in 1998.

Hepatitis and end-stage liver disease, however, emerged as an important cause of sickness and death in this population. In 1995 hepatitis and liver disease accounted for only 4 percent of deaths, but two years later the number rose to 14 percent!

Resources: For more information about the current treatment for HIV/AIDS, contact the following hotlines and information services:

CDC National HIV/AIDS Hotline: 1-800-342-2437 (English); 1-800-344-7432 (Spanish); 1-800-243-7889 (TDD)

CDC National Sexually Transmitted Diseases (STD) Hotline: 1-800-227-8922

CDC website: www.cdc.gov

Complications of HAART Therapy

Effect of Hepatitis C (HCV) Infection on HIV. Although there is no evidence for a direct effect of hepatitis C on HIV, the major clinical issue is clear: Hepatitis C can complicate therapy of HIV. Currently, the Federal Drug Administration has licensed more than 13 drugs for treatment of HIV in the United States. Nearly all of these medications, but in particular the protease inhibitors, are metabolized in some way by the liver.

As liver disease due to hepatitis C progresses from hepatitis to cirrhosis, the liver is less able to metabolize these compounds. Changes in liver function may make it necessary to change the drugs used and the doses of individual drugs. In addition, the anti-HIV drugs may be toxic to the liver. Instances of liver enzyme elevations, jaundice, and even fatal cases of severe liver toxicity from anti-HIV medications have occurred.

I had never heard of hepatitis C before. I figured I already had HIV-AIDS, so what difference did hepatitis C make? My doctors pulled me off all my AIDS meds twice because my liver enzymes went crazy. My whole body went crazy. I was nauseous and vomiting.

Turned out I had a fungus in my esophagus from not being on the medications. I'm sick if I take the medicine and sick if I don't.

Anna

Effect of HIV Infection on Hepatitis C. As described in preceding chapters, a chronic hepatitis C patient's own immune system can injure the liver as the immune system tries to destroy infected liver cells (immune-mediated injury). In contrast, after a transplant the viral levels are very high due to the use of immunosuppressive medications, and the virus itself destroys liver cells. Thus, HIV infection, which destroys components of the immune response, may either slow or accelerate liver disease due to hepatitis C.

Because HIV infection affects the immune system, it might impair a patient's immune response to hepatitis C and result in higher levels of the hepatitis C virus. One French study compared 75 patients with hepatitis C to 75 patients co-infected with hepatitis C and HIV. Co-infected patients were more likely to have positive HCV-RNA in their blood, and their HCV-RNA levels were significantly higher. However, the level of HCV-RNA did not correlate with CD4 count (a measure of the degree of immune deficiency), p24 antigen levels (a specific HIV protein), or HIV-RNA level.

In contrast, a German study of 21 co-infected hemophiliacs and 22 hemophiliacs with isolated hepatitis C failed to show a difference in HCV-RNA viral levels between these two groups. Another study retrospectively examined stored serum for HCV-RNA levels in groups of hemophiliacs infected with hepatitis C. Those who subsequently developed HIV experienced a significant increase in HCV-RNA level, which correlated with the reduction in CD4 count.

One fear is that these drugs may actually accelerate the progression of hepatitis C to cirrhosis and therefore compromise the effectiveness of therapy against HIV. Researchers examined this issue in a study of HAART therapy in 51 patients with "HCV-related chronic liver disease." HAART therapy was associated with an increase in HCV-RNA viral load and elevations in liver enzymes (AST/ALT) within one to three months of starting treatment. Liver biopsies revealed liver cell injury and inflammation. Seven patients were taken off HAART due to signs of liver failure. This effect was mainly due to HAART because a much smaller number of patients not on HAART (four out of 148) experienced symptoms of liver failure. However, the worsened liver inflammation noted early in HAART therapy had largely subsided by nine months on HAART. Additional research is needed in this area.

A recent study examined the development of abnormal liver tests after 394 HIV patients began HAART treatment. Seven percent were co-infected with hepatitis B and 14 percent had hepatitis C. The risk of developing abnormal liver tests was greater in HIV patients who had chronic hepatitis (37 percent in co-infected patients vs. 12 percent in HIV patients without either HBV or HCV). Although inconclusive, these data suggest that the immune deficiency caused by HIV may promote hepatitis C viral replication and potentially hasten the progression of liver disease.

Does HIV Co-Infection Affect the Rate of Progression of Liver Disease?

The CDC has reported that the percentage of HIV patients with death due to liver disease steadily increased from 1987 to 1997. According to data from the U.S. National Vital Statistics System, the percent of death certificates listing "sequelae (consequences) of chronic liver disease" increased from 1.3 percent in 1987, to 2.2 percent in 1995, to 3.5 percent in 1997.

Further analysis of death certificates indicated that liver disease caused, contributed, or was secondarily involved in approximately 10 percent of all deaths in 1997. Patients dying with a diagnosis of chronic hepatitis C increased from 0.9 percent in 1995 to 2.3 percent in 1997 (tests for hepatitis C were not available until 1990). Patients dying with a diagnosis of chronic hepatitis B increased from 0.5 percent in 1987, to 0.8 percent in 1995, to 1.3 percent in 1997.

The observed increase in deaths related to "sequelae of chronic liver disease" exceeded the expected frequency by 46 percent. It is not known whether the increase in mortality rate was due to use of HAART medications, increased activity of hepatitis viruses, or reflected the natural progression of hepatitis B and C occurring in HIV patients who now live longer.

Only a few studies have examined the association between HIV infection and acceleration in liver disease related to hepatitis C. One large retrospective series from Spain examined 547 patients who acquired hepatitis C by blood-borne routes and found that 116 of these patients were co-infected with HIV. The researchers observed that co-infected people took less time to develop cirrhosis. At ten years of HCV infection, 14.9 percent of co-infected patients had cirrhosis, compared to only 2.6 percent of those infected only with hepatitis C.

A French series of 210 patients with hepatitis C, 60 of whom were co-infected with HIV, suggested that the incidence of cirrhosis was 3.5 times higher in co-infected patients. Another study from Spain examined liver histology and found that co-infected patients had more severe liver inflammation and later stages of fibrosis.

None of these studies were controlled or randomized, so it is not clear whether liver disease is truly more aggressive in this population. However, these limited studies do suggest that hepatitis C-related liver disease may accelerate under the influence of immune deficiency. We need more careful investigation in controlled trials.

Antiviral Therapy of Hepatitis C in Patients Co-Infected with HIV

The first published experience in treating HCV/HIV patients appeared in 1992. Twelve patients with HIV/HCV had documented abnormal ALT levels for more than six months, were HCV antibody positive, and had chronic active hepatitis (two had cirrhosis). The patients were treated with interferon–alfa monotherapy at a variety of doses ranging from one to five million units (1 to 5 MU) three times a week (tiw) for four to six months. Four patients (33 percent) had a complete response (normalization of ALT) on treatment, but only one sustained the response six months after treatment.

Another study, published in 1993, treated 14 patients with HIV/HCV (one cirrhotic) with nine million units (9 MU) daily for three months followed by 9 MU three times a week (tiw) for three months, 6 MU tiw for three months, and then 3 MU tiw for three months. Only nine patients completed the therapy, but five of the nine were complete responders according to their ALT levels. Only three of the five had negative HCV-RNA viral levels, and four of the five sustained the response once treatment was stopped.

The largest published study of interferon monotherapy involved 119 patients (90 HIV positive, 29 HIV negative) treated with 5 MU tiw for three months. Nonresponders were then dropped from therapy, and responders continued on therapy for an additional six months at 3 MU tiw. Eighty HIV patients and 27 non-HIV patients completed the course of treatment; 32.5 percent and 37 percent were negative for HCV-RNA at the end of treatment, respectively. Sustained responses after discontinuation of treatment were not described. CD4 counts greater than 500 and low levels of HCV-RNA were predictors of response in co-infected patients.

In summary, monotherapy with interferon may yield a response rate in HIV infected patients similar to non–HIV patients. A number of trials evaluating the safety and effectiveness of combination therapy are currently underway. As of this writing, the results have not yet been published. Physicians must weigh the potential benefits of therapy against side effects and the ability of the patient to tolerate the drug.

Are New Treatments on the Horizon for Co-Infected Patients? Currently, trials are underway to determine whether pegylated interferon plus ribavirin will improve the rate of HCV clearance. Other possibilites for therapy include thymosin–alpha-1, HCV-specific protease inhibitors, HCV-specific helicase inhibitors, and others (see Chapters 8, 9, and 14). Your doctor may be able to tell you if you are a candidate for participating in trials of any of these therapies.

Resources: For more information about treatment and trials, call the following hotlines and information services:

AIDS Treatment Information Service (ATIS): 1-800-448-0440
Project Inform: 1-800-822-7422
Aids Clinical Trials Information Service: 1-800-TRIALS-A

Co-Infection with Hepatitis B

> The worst thing for me is the fatigue. Although everyone with hep-
> atitis seems to suffer to some degree, my experience has been extreme.
> My doctor thinks that maybe because I have two viruses, B and C, my
> body fights twice as hard and causes me to be increasingly more tired.
>
> *Mel*

Co-infection with hepatitis B and C, each of which independently
damages the liver, results in greater liver damage and more rapid progression to cirrhosis. Current estimates suggest that 33 percent of
patients with chronic hepatitis C are co-infected with hepatitis B. Two-
thirds of patients have isolated hepatitis B core antibody, and one-third
lack all serologic markers for hepatitis B but have positive HBV-DNA.
Although co-infection may suppress rates of viral replication, and levels
of HCV-RNA may be relatively lower, liver damage is increased.

A recent case-control study confirmed the reciprocal relationship
between inhibition of viral replication and liver damage. Co-infected
patients, despite lower viral replication, were more likely to have either
moderate to severe chronic hepatitis or cirrhosis. Co-infected patients
may also have a greater risk of developing hepatocellular carcinoma, in
other words, liver cancer (see Chapter 11).

In general, therapy is recommended for co-infected patients. Doctors often try to determine which of the two viruses dominate the other
(in terms of contributing to the liver injury) in order to choose therapy.
This decision is often based upon the tests for hepatitis B. The patient
with positive HBV-DNA and hepatitis B e antigen may have dominant
hepatitis B and warrant lamivudine or daily interferon in relatively high
doses for four to six months. The patient who is negative for HBV-DNA
and hepatitis B e antigen may have dominant hepatitis C and warrant
combination therapy plus ribavirin for up to one year.

With me, the C is the active virus and the B is apparently rather inert. I was so tired and irritable, I had to quit night school—and my goal was to finish college before my kids. When I tried to go back, there was no brain left. I had migraines, joint pain, arthritis.

I read that if you have B as well, the hepatitis is worse, so I decided to try treatment. I made my husband promise not to leave me if I went on interferon. The first night, my husband and I sat on the couch and waited for the side effects. We both fell asleep.

When I woke up, I had no joint pain. It's been eight months, and I feel better on interferon. My labs are good. The C is undetectable.

Ina

My son, a hemophiliac, is co-infected. He got non-A, non-B hepatitis at age 1. Later they diagnosed it as hepatitis C. He got it from the clotting factor they gave him to stop the bleeds. Today they heat the clotting factor to kill viruses.

He's 19 now and more concerned about being contagious with the hepatitis B in regard to his social life. His doctor started him on six months of combo therapy for the C but with daily doses of interferon to hit the B hard. In July he tested negative for the first time ever for hepatitis B surface antigens. And he tested less than 200 for a hepatitis C viral load after a six-month treatment of daily interferon and ribavirin!

Sophie

Recent evidence suggests that ribavirin may also be effective against hepatitis B. This observation, coupled with the emergence of pegylated interferons, suggests that the best future therapy for co-infected patients may be the combination of pegylated interferon with ribavirin. Regardless of choice of therapy, effectiveness must be determined with PCR tests to measure both HBV-DNA and HCV-RNA (see Chapter 2). Subsequent treatment should be tailored to the outcome of the first course.

In clinical practice, a liver biopsy does not help to determine the dominance of one infection over the other, because the histologic (cell) changes with hepatitis B and C are similar. Research tests (including immunohistochemical examination and molecular studies of biopsy material) may be able to distinguish the dominant infection, but their clinical usefulness is not defined.

I didn't have a clue I was sick until I had a bleed. I was in the hospital eight or nine days. When the tests came back, they were positive for hepatitis B and C. My biopsy showed I only had 25 percent liver function. I had cirrhosis so bad, the doctor said I was a candidate for a transplant. I had active hepatitis C and inactive hepatitis B. The fear was that after the transplant, because of the immunosuppressive drugs and the surgery, the B could flare up.

Juliet

Resource: For more information on hepatitis B, contact the organizations listed in the Resources section at the end of this book and the Hepatitis B Foundation, 700 E. Butler Ave., Doylestown, PA 18901-2697; phone: 215-489-4900; email: info@hepb.org; website: www.hepb.org.

Resource: For an online hepatitis B support group, contact the Hepatitis B Information and Support List: http://www. geocities.com/ Heartland/Estates/9350/hblist.html. To subscribe, send a blank email to: hepatitis-b-on@mail-list.com.

Resource: For up-to-the-minute research reports, subscribe to the free Hepatitis B Research List by sending a blank email to: HBV_Research-on@mail-list.com. The research bulletins from 1998 to the current year are archived at http://dispatch.mail-list.com/archives/ hbv_research and can be accessed by an easy search engine.

Resource: Everson, Gregory T., M.D., and Hedy Weinberg. *Living with Hepatitis B: A Survivor's Guide.* New York: Hatherleigh Press, 2001.

Liver Transplantation

Hepatitis C patients co-infected with hepatitis B are considered candidates for liver transplantation using the same criteria established for isolated hepatitis C. Transplantation for patients co-infected with HIV is controversial and there are only limited reports from a few centers.

Transplantation before HAART. Before HAART physicians refused to consider HIV-infected patients for liver transplantation for the following reasons:

1. The immunosuppressive medications used after transplantation to prevent rejection of the donor liver would have further compromised the HIV-induced immune deficiency and increased the risk of serious life-threatening infection or malignancy.
2. HIV patients typically had ongoing infections, malignancies, or other illnesses that prohibited transplantation.
3. HIV patients would likely have died of HIV-related complications despite liver transplantation, thereby wasting a donor liver.

Anecdotal reports of liver transplantation in HIV-infected patients before the era of HAART therapy indicated that HIV patients continued to have HIV after the transplant. They experienced a predictable downhill course. Therefore, many transplant centers disqualified HIV patients from receiving liver transplants. With effective treatment now available, many transplant centers are reconsidering HIV patients with cirrhosis for liver transplantation. Current Medicare and Medicaid guidelines regarding HIV are under review and modification.

> *I'm really worried. If I get cirrhosis, they won't give me a transplant because I have AIDS. That will be it. The end. No options.*
>
> *At my hepatitis C support group they told me to take it one step at a time. First, I need a liver biopsy and a PCR viral load test. But I can't stop my mind from racing ahead and obsessing.*
>
> *The only thing that keeps me going is God.*
>
> *Reuben*

Transplantation after HAART. HAART therapy may make liver transplantation an option for HIV-infected patients. HAART therapy has been so effective that the projected life span for an HIV-infected individual now extends from less than five years to more than 20 years. Patients co-infected with HIV/HCV may remain stable in terms of the complications of their immune deficiency only to experience significant liver disease, liver failure, and the need for liver transplantation.

At the University of Colorado Health Sciences Center, deaths of HIV-infected patients in 1997 were nearly as often due to hepatitis and end-stage liver disease as to opportunistic infections or malignancy. In fact, deaths due to liver disease surpassed deaths due to advanced HIV, which includes AIDS wasting syndrome and dementia. Although many centers performing liver transplants now are revisiting the question, there is still great reluctance to perform liver transplants in HIV patients.

Summary

We are just beginning to address the growing problem of co-infection of hepatitis C patients with either HIV or hepatitis B. As patients with HIV/AIDS live decades longer due to new antiviral treatments, many of them will have to deal with hepatitis C treatment decisions as well. These are complicated issues because HIV/AIDS therapies affect the liver, and hepatitis C therapies affect the immune system.

My hope is that new studies, advances in drug therapy, and controlled research projects will yield more information about all of these viruses. Then physicians and patients can work together to make thoughtful plans for treatment and to offer more options to patients affected by both HIV/AIDS and hepatitis B and C.

A journey of a thousand miles must begin with a single step.

Lao-tzu

Reference

1. S. Johnson, A. Hageman, H. Wing, M. Grodesky, N. Bathurst, P. Romfh, W. Williams. Effect of Antiretroviral Therapy on Clinical Outcomes and Cost in a University-Based HIV/AIDS Program: 1995-1997. Abstract 42211, 12th World AIDS Conference, Geneva, Switzerland, June 23-July 3, 1998.

13

CHILDREN WITH HEPATITIS C

A Growing Problem

Five years ago I donated blood. I got a letter with a box checked off: hepatitis C. I never had any symptoms, and the doctors think I got infected from transfusions I had years ago.

I really wasn't alarmed until they tested my husband and my three kids. My youngest—my 3-year-old baby girl—was the only one with hepatitis C. She had slightly elevated enzymes and her biopsy showed a little bit of scarring. The doctors want to give her interferon.

What do I do? She's so little. If I have hepatitis C, it's my problem, and I did it to myself. I'll deal with whatever treatment I have to. But to make the decision for my child is much, much harder.

Betsy

WHEN CHILDREN HAVE a serious infection, like hepatitis C, it affects the whole family. Parents nurture their children through life-threatening diseases only to learn that blood transfusions (before screening tests ensured the safety of the blood supply) gave them hepatitis C. Mothers feel a profound sense of guilt if they passed the virus to their babies.

> *I'm a nurse, so I was stuck and splashed on for years. In 1995 I found out I had hepatitis C. Seven years before, I had given birth to my first baby—a little boy, Andy. He never had any symptoms or signs of hepatitis C, but I got scared and had both my kids tested—sure I was paranoid. Andy's test was positive.*
>
> *I was devastated, guilty. I felt it was my fault. My husband never accused me but said, "You were not careful enough in the operating room." I felt terrible.*
>
> Shanna

Researchers are just beginning to study treatment in children, so current information is often vague and indefinite. And that adds to a parent's anxiety. As a parent, you feel concerned about your family—and you're concerned about yourself, too, if you're ill with hepatitis C.

> *I can't continue raising my kids and working. I lie in the bathtub and bawl. My kids are active, and I need downtime. It's hard when you have hepatitis C and one of your kids has it too.*
>
> *Sometimes I plug in a movie for them so I can lie down. I can hardly move. I feel like a terrible mother. I always said I'd never park them in front of a TV.*
>
> Janice

How do children get hepatitis C? Although a child may become infected when the mother passes the infection to her baby at birth (the vertical route), some children acquired hepatitis C from exposure to blood or blood products (through treatment of conditions such as congenital heart disease, malignancies, leukemia, hemophilia, and other illnesses) before blood was screened for the virus.

Adolescents may acquire hepatitis C through exposure to infected blood or through intravenous drug use. This age group has its own problems with care and management of hepatitis C. However, issues regarding diagnosis, medical treatment, progression of liver disease, and transplantation are probably similar to the adult population, and I refer you to those topics in previous chapters.

   Note: Discussions and recommendations in this chapter are meant as guidelines. Please consult your pediatrician, or your pediatric gastroenterologist or hepatologist regarding specific issues in treatment and management.

   Here are the topics we'll cover:

- Overview
- Does Your Baby Have Hepatitis C?
   Antibody Testing
   HCV-RNA Assays
   Can Infection Be Prevented?
- Should Women with Hepatitis C Avoid Pregnancy or Breastfeeding?
- Can Your Child Participate in Regular Activities?
   Disclosure: To Tell or Not To Tell
   Chronic Disease and Your Family
   Resources for Children
- The Course of the Infection in Children
- Monitoring Children with Hepatitis C
   Liver Biopsy
   Blood Draws and Biopsies/Practical Suggestions
- Treatment
   Interferon Therapy
   Interferon Plus Ribavirin
   Pegylated Interferon
   Giving Injections
   Future Therapy
   Post-Treatment Follow-Up

Overview

Hepatitis C in children is a growing problem. According to the American Liver Foundation, one of every 500 children (0.2 percent) between the ages of 6 and 11 is chronically infected by hepatitis C. In children between the ages of 12 and 19, one of every 250 (0.4 percent) is infected.

   Most transmissions of hepatitis C to an infant occur during delivery when the infant may be exposed to the mother's blood. Prior to 1992 a common route of acquisition of hepatitis C, even in young children, was previous exposure to blood or blood products through transfusion. Screening with current tests has virtually eliminated this mode of transmission.

A mother with hepatitis C may transmit the virus to her infant at the birth of the newborn. The risk of this type of transmission correlates with the presence of HCV-RNA viral load in the mother's blood at the time of delivery. Mothers co-infected with HIV and hepatitis C are even more likely to transmit hepatitis C to their newborn.

Several studies have found that when mothers have hepatitis C, the chance that the infant will acquire the virus is approximately 6 percent. In contrast, the likelihood of transmission increases to more than 15 percent when mothers are co-infected with hepatitis C and HIV. The increased risk of transmission in HIV-positive mothers may be related to the relatively higher concentration of HCV-RNA in their blood. Given the fact that these infants are at risk, the U.S. Public Health Service recommends that all children born of hepatitis C-infected mothers be tested for the virus.

Does Your Baby Have Hepatitis C?

Antibody Testing. Hepatitis C antibodies in the mother's blood cross the placental barrier and are detected in the baby's blood. This movement of the mother's antibodies to the baby is called passive transfer and does not mean that the virus itself has transferred to the baby. Hepatitis C antibodies do not protect the baby, and the infant may or may not develop hepatitis C infection.

Passively acquired antibodies usually persist for 6 to 12 months and never beyond 15 months. If the baby undergoes antibody testing 15 months or more after delivery and the HCV antibody is positive, it is likely that the infant has been infected with hepatitis C.

HCV-RNA Assays. Because of the problems with antibody testing, most hepatologists favor measuring viral load with an HCV-RNA assay, such as a PCR assay (see Chapter 2), to determine whether the infant is actively infected with hepatitis C. In most cases, truly infected infants will test positive for HCV-RNA within two months of birth. HCV-RNA will remain positive as long as the virus continues to replicate and persist in the child.

Can Infection Be Prevented? We don't have an effective antiviral strategy to prevent infection of the newborn. Immune serum globulin, even when it contains a high concentration of the antibody against hepatitis C, does not prevent transmission, and no one has studied pre-emptive use of antiviral therapy (interferon, etc). In addition, it probably makes little sense to expose all babies to the risks of gamma globulin therapy or interferon when the vast majority will not acquire hepatitis C.

For these reasons physicians recommend simply monitoring for hepatitis C. Minimum testing requirements include measurement of the hepatitis C antibody 12 months after delivery. Hepatitis C infection could be detected earlier by measuring HCV-RNA viral load one to two months after birth. Umbilical cord blood should not be used for testing of either the hepatitis C antibody or the HCV-RNA viral load because it may be contaminated with maternal blood.

Should Women with Hepatitis C Avoid Pregnancy or Breastfeeding?

The decision to proceed with childbearing is personal and individual. Most experts in this field conclude that women should not avoid preg-nancy simply because they have hepatitis C, even though there is the potential risk of transmitting the virus to their infant. In otherwise healthy mothers, 94 percent of offspring will not acquire hepatitis C; only 6 percent get the infection, and the course of hepatitis C in these infants has been clinically mild in the majority of cases. However, the long-term consequences of chronic HCV infection acquired vertically has not been studied.

Nonetheless, parents must realize that there is a risk and that we don't completely understand the long-term consequences of hepatitis C in an infant who acquires the virus. Some infants may develop hepatitis, progress to cirrhosis over several years, and may even require liver trans-plantation in the future. In addition, all infants who become chronic car-riers may be at some risk for developing liver cancer—although we don't have any data on this yet.

Studies have examined the risk of the newborn acquiring hepatitis C related to the type of delivery. Early studies showed that the risk was similar whether the baby was delivered vaginally or by Cesarian section (C-section), and the U.S. Public Health Service has not recommended Cesarian section as the routine method of delivery. However, a recent study showed that delivery by elective Cesarean section prior to mem-brane rupture was associated with a lower transmission risk than either vaginal or emergent Cesarean section delivery. Additional studies are needed before elective Cesarian section can be recommended.

In addition, there is little evidence that breastfeeding increases the risk of transmitting hepatitis C. In one study, the number of cases of hepatitis C in breastfed and bottle-fed infants born of mothers infected with hepatitis C was the same (4 percent). Epidemiological studies indicate that breastfeeding has not been definitely shown to transmit hepatitis C to infants. Given these data, the U. S. Public Health Service does not currently restrict breastfeeding for mothers with hepatitis C. Of course, women should discuss this decision with their physicians and pediatricians.

However, recent information suggests that infants who are breastfed and whose mothers have active symptoms of hepatitis C may be at increased risk. Mothers with active, aggressive hepatitis C (for example, jaundice) should avoid or abstain from breastfeeding if their nipples are cracked or bleeding. Always consult with your doctor.

Can Your Child Participate in Regular Activities?

Hepatitis C is not spread by casual contact, and children with the virus may participate in all regular activities, including school, play, day care, childcare, extracurricular activities, and sports. One exception would be the child who has active skin wounds and sores. The official American Academy of Pediatrics (AAP) recommendation is that the open wound be completely covered with a secure bandage or dressing before participation in the activity.

Tell your child that he or she cannot give hepatitis C to friends, classmates, family, or other acquaintances by sneezing, coughing, holding, hugging, or kissing; by sharing food, water, eating utensils or drinking glasses; or by any other casual contact. The Centers for Disease Control guidelines don't disqualify anyone from school unless they show aggressive behavior, such as biting or scratching.

Hepatitis C can be spread by blood exposure, so cuts or abrasions should be carefully cleaned and bandaged to avoid contact with other children. In addition, the child should be told to avoid putting his or her fingers in other children's mouths (in order to prevent possible biting), sharing toothbrushes or razor blades, and making other contact with open sores or wounds.

Parents will be pleased to know that in December 2000, the AAP announced that athletes with HIV, HBV, or HCV should be allowed to

participate in all sports and that doctors should maintain patient confidentiality. The AAP policy statement states that there is a "very low
probability" that these infections would be transmitted among young
athletes. The AAP recommends that athletic programs use Occupational
Safety and Health Administration (OSHA) Universal Precautions and
inform students and parents that there is a "very small but finite risk" of
a blood-borne infection.

Resource: To read the entire policy statement, go to the AAP website: www.aap.org/policy/re9821.html.

Disclosure: To Tell or Not To Tell. One of the major problems
you face as a parent is disclosure. It's important to tell doctors and dentists about your child's condition, but do you tell the daycare facility, the
school, caregivers, friends?

"There is a disparity between the ideal and the real situation," says
Marjanne Claassen, R.N., M.S., C.N.S., Clinical Nurse Specialist and
Pediatric Liver Center Nurse Coordinator in the Section of Pediatric
Gastroenterology, Hepatology and Nutrition at The Children's Hospital
in Denver, Colorado. "The approach in schools is to use standard precautions. The ideal is that every staff member will deal with every child's
blood in the same protective way. The OSHA standards require that all
blood is assumed to be contaminated. Therefore, the school worker must
assume that there are germs in everybody's blood, and of course with
any blood-borne illness most children have it well before anyone knows
they have it.

"Protective Personal Equipment (PPE—disposable protective
gloves) is usually all that's needed. Because of standard precautions, the
family has no legal obligation to tell anyone a child's diagnosis. That's the
ideal.

"The reality is that the parent usually chooses to tell the school. I
recommend that families notify the professional registered nurse in
charge of their child's school. A registered nurse understands the issues
of confidentiality and will be prepared to handle questions as they come
up."

"Be knowledgeable yourself," says Nancy Butler-Simon, M.S.,
R.N., C.N.S., C.P.N.P., Advanced Practice Nurse at Denver Children's
Hospital's Pediatric General Clinical Research Center. "Be right up
front with the school nurse. Have a script. Educate people. The school
nurse can help you do that. Panic is the most contagious thing on this

planet; deal with it by teaching others. Nip anxiety in the bud with knowledge."

Aside from school, parents and children must also decide what friends to inform and how. Parents must find the balance between secrecy and privacy. It's important to communicate that hepatitis C is not transmitted casually, but is a blood-borne infection.

My biggest fear is they'll label him and say, "Stay away from him. He's got that virus!" But as my mother says, "Things happen. The dear Lord doesn't give you any more than you can handle."

My husband and I always tell the parents of our children's friends in case something should happen. The parents say, "Oh, I'll keep an eye out." It's not like they don't invite her over. They say, "Don't worry about it."

My mom tells my friends' moms what to do if I cut myself. She tells them to put gloves on and not touch my blood because I have hepatitis C.

Everyone in the family knows. The daycare providers knew when she was little. Nothing has ever had to be done to treat her differently.

My daughter doesn't tell her friends. She doesn't want to feel like she has the plague. She does know she needs to be careful with her blood. From the beginning I talked to her. "Don't let them use your toothbrush or razor. Don't use theirs. Put a bandage on a cut yourself."

My brother, Tommy's uncle, got really angry at me when I decided to delay treatment for Tommy. He yelled at me and grabbed my arm— my own brother. "You're killing him!" he said.

Tommy had no symptoms, and it was a hard call, but the hardest thing of all was the lack of support in my own family.

It helps that I have hepatitis C too. I wouldn't know how to deal with my 7-year-old daughter otherwise. I know what she's feeling when she comes to me with a concern.

My husband has to use gloves to help us clean up if my daughter or I are bleeding. He felt bad. I said, "Just do it. Just put them on."

As children approach adolescence, parents should discuss decisions about future behaviors. Ideally, the topics of body piercing, tattooing, illegal drugs, and safe sex will be introduced in the context of family values when children are young. Pre-adolescence is an opportunity to make youngsters aware that you can not only give diseases such as hepatitis C and AIDS, you can also get these illnesses from these exposures.

In summary, says Claassen, "Think carefully before you share your child's diagnosis. Balance responsibility with caution and with making your child's life as normal as possible. You don't want a big red 'H' on your child's head."

Resource: Many organizations offer information to parents. Some also provide sample letters that can be given to schools. Contact Parents of Kids with Infectious Diseases (PKIDs) and other groups listed in the Resources section at the end of this book.

Resource: The *Pediatric Hepatitis Report,* co-funded by the CDC and Parents of Kids with Infectious Diseases (PKIDs), is available online at the PKIDs website: www.pkids.org. The report covers hepatitis A through E, the latest treatment options, liver tests, children's civil rights, how to tell others about your child's disease, how to tell your child, and more. You may obtain a hard copy for a fee by contacting the organization. See the Resources section at the end of this book.

Chronic Disease and Your Family. Hepatitis C affects everyone in the family—in positive as well as negative ways (see Chapter 5). What family friends do you tell, and when do you tell them? How do you deal with brothers and sisters who worry about the sick sibling but may be jealous over the extra attention paid to the child with hepatitis C?

Another big issue is body image. Children don't like to feel different. Sometimes, even if they have no symptoms of hepatitis C, they may think they look different. Talk to your children. Let them tell you their fears and reassure them. Above all, your child needs to know that hepatitis C is a medical condition, not a reason to feel ashamed.

Worry? No, I don't. Not really. My mom doesn't have really bad hepatitis C.

When my sister or mom gets hurt, we have to wear gloves. But mostly I don't talk about it. Sometimes something comes up, and you have to explain what it is, like when kids are talking about other diseases.

I tell them it's a sickness, and it affects your liver sometimes. For my sister, it does. It can kill you, but it doesn't most often. And sometimes they ask me questions I can't answer.

Hannah, age 9

Chronic disease is a strain, emotionally and financially. Your pediatrician and local children's hospital have resources to help you: social workers, specialists in financial matters, nurses, and doctors who've dealt with the same problems you're facing.

Talking to others, either informally or in support groups, can help you keep your perspective.

Resource: Contact the PKIDs Support List for parents (kids are encouraged to participate). Also, access the PKIDs research archives: www.pkids.org.

Resources for Children. The organizations listed in Resources at the back of this book provide avenues to support groups, online chat groups, videotapes, research archives, and educational packets. Your local children's hospital library also is a good source of information.

On Healthy Eating. A low-fat, balanced, healthy diet is appropriate for people with liver disease (see Chapter 5). Note: Parents of children with cirrhosis should consult their doctors about dietary restrictions. For a free copy of the colorful *Tips for Using the Food Guide Pyramid for Young Children 2 to 6 Years Old* (with recipes), contact the U.S. Department of Agriculture, Center for Nutrition Policy and Promotion: 202-606-8000; website: www.usda.gov/cnpp.

On Hepatitis.

Aronson, Virginia. *Everything You Need to Know About Hepatitis.* New York: Rosen Publishing Group, 2000 (middle school, high school).

"Hepachallenge." The American Digestive Health Foundation offers this free interactive computer game (on CD-ROM), which deals with prevention of hepatitis (adolescents). To order, call 1-800-668-5237.

Silverstein, Alvin, Virginia & Robert. *Hepatitis.* Springfield: Enslow Publishers, 1994 (middle school, high school).

Weinberg, Hedy and Shira Shump with Gregory T. Everson, M.D. *My Mom Has Hepatitis C*. Long Island City: Hatherleigh Press, 2000 (preschool, elementary).

On Issues of Chronic Illness.

Band-aids and Blackboards. A colorful website about growing up with medical problems with areas for kids, teens, and adults; website: http://funrsc.fairfield.edu/~ifleitas/contents.html.

Heegard, Marge. *When Someone Has a Very Serious Illness*. Mpls.: Woodland Press, 1991 (workbook for preschool and elementary).

Huegel, Kelly. *Young People and Chronic Illness (True Stories, Help, and Hope)*. Mpls.: Free Spirit, 1998 (middle school, high school).

LeVert Suzanne. *Face to Face with Chronic Illness*. New York: Messner/Simon & Schuster, 1993 (high school).

Moe, Barbara. *Coping with Chronic Illness*. New York: Rosen Publishing Group, 1992 (middle school, high school).

On Children Facing Liver Transplants:

Murphy-Melas, Elizabeth. *Pennies, Nickels & Dimes*. Santa Fe: Health Press, 1999.

Ribal, Lizzy. *Lizzy Gets a New Liver/Lizzy Tiene un Hígado Nuevo*. Louisville: Bridge Resources, 1997.

Shadow Buddies. A website that offers condition-specific dolls for your child, including one for liver transplant patients (complete with hospital gown, "Y" incision, and Hickman catheter), with a link to Shadow Buddies Foundation; website: www.shadowbuddies.com.

The Course of the Infection in Children

We don't yet know the natural history or course of hepatitis C in children who acquire the disease vertically from mother to infant at the time of delivery. The rate of development of long-term consequences, such as cirrhosis, liver failure, or liver cancer, is unknown. Persistent infection with hepatitis C may occur in greater than 70 percent of infected newborns. Most infants with hepatitis C have a benign course, even though the majority does demonstrate mild elevations in liver enzymes. Few (less than 15 percent) exhibit more severe liver injury including clinical jaundice. Occasionally, a child will have more aggressive hepatitis and progressive fibrosis.

One recent study examined liver biopsies performed in 74 boys and 35 girls with chronic hepatitis C, ages 4 to 14. All were positive for HCV antibody or had HCV-RNA in blood samples, and all had persistently elevated ALT (greater than 1.5 times normal) for at least six months prior to the biopsy. Results were compared to biopsies from 120 adults.

Most of these children had acquired hepatitis C by exposure to blood or blood products (85 percent) and only 11 percent were vertically transmitted from mother to infant. When researchers studied the liver biopsies under a microscope, they discovered that children had milder degrees of inflammation and lower histologic stages compared to adults. This finding implies a slower progression of disease in children. In fact, none of the biopsies in children demonstrated cirrhosis. However, additional controlled studies to define rates of progression of hepatitis C in children are needed.

NOTE: All patients with underlying liver disease, including hepatitis C, should receive the hepatitis A and hepatitis B vaccines. Please consult your pediatrician, pediatric gastroenterologist, or hepatologist. The hepatitis A vaccine is recommended for children over 2 years of age.

Resource: If you can't afford vaccination shots or don't know where to get them, contact your city, county, or state health department, or call the Centers for Disease Control's Immunization Information Hotline at 1-800-232-2522. For Spanish language inquiries, call 1-800-232-0233.

Monitoring Children with Hepatitis C

According to Michael R. Narkewicz, M.D., Medical Director of The Pediatric Liver Center and Liver Transplant Program at The Children's Hospital in Denver and Associate Professor in Pediatrics at the University of Colorado Medical School, Hewit Andrews Chair in Pediatric Liver Disease, there are no standard recommendations. "Here at The Pediatric Liver Center, our recommendation is that the child should have liver blood tests performed once or twice a year (more frequently if the liver blood tests are abnormal), alpha-fetoprotein (tumor marker) every six months, and an ultrasound at a minimum of every two years or if the alpha-fetoprotein is rising.

"There are currently no FDA-approved treatments for hepatitis C in children. There are reports of children who received treatment for chronic hepatitis C with interferon. In general, the indications for considering potential treatment are persistently abnormal liver blood tests or evidence of liver disease on physical exam with an abnormal liver biopsy."

Liver Biopsy.

I was kind of sore after my biopsy, but I watched lots of movies. The nurses moved the bed up and down. And I got spaghetti, pizza, chocolate pudding, and JELL-O®!

Haley, age 6

"I think liver biopsy is mandatory before deciding on a course of treatment," says Dr. Narkewicz, "because it tells us how much scarring has occurred in the liver and makes sure that the abnormal blood tests are the result of hepatitis C and not some other unsuspected liver disease.

"We do all our liver biopsies using the needle biopsy technique under sedation or anesthesia to make it more comfortable for the child, less anxiety-provoking, and to minimize risks. It is either a day surgical procedure or involves a short overnight stay. The major risk is bleeding, so we always assess children's blood clotting before a liver biopsy. The risk of significant bleeding in pediatric liver biopsies is about 1 percent."

Blood Draws and Biopsies/Practical Suggestions.

My older daughter, Leigh, was in kindergarten and having a really hard time. She was so worried that something was wrong with her sister, Tammy, that she cried a lot and had nightmares.

I finally learned to schedule Tammy's blood tests when Leigh was somewhere else. The blood tests didn't bother Tammy that much, but Leigh couldn't stand watching the needles, the blood.

So now Tammy and I get our blood drawn together.

Mother of
Leigh and Tammy

When I was little, I couldn't stand to have my sister hurt from the blood draws. So I would cry too. I couldn't watch. I'd put my face against the wall and cry and Tammy, who was only 2, would say, "That didn't hurt."

Tammy's sister, Leigh

When a child has hepatitis C, parents frequently have to prepare their child for painful procedures, such as blood draws and biopsies. According to Butler-Simon, emotional pain and physical pain are equally challenging and often inseparable. Doctors and nurses often underestimate pain, but parents know their children best and should be advocates on their behalf.

In 1996 Laura's enzymes shot up into the 70s. They did a hepatitis screen, and sure enough, she had it. It meant constant blood tests. She had one experience where they stuck her five times. She'd scream and carry on. It was traumatic.

Then a nurse told us about this topical anesthetic cream, EMLA® Cream. You put a pretty fair amount over the vein and put a clear dressing on it. You can even use that sticky wrap you cover food with. Keep the cream in place for an hour. It makes life easier for kids afraid of a needle.

Mary

Here are some of Butler-Simon's practical suggestions:

- Use EMLA® Cream to numb the area before a blood draw. Left on the skin for an hour, it will numb the area up to a half-inch deep.
- Give Tylenol® beforehand (size- and age-recommended dosage).
- Prepare the child beforehand, using language and concepts that are developmentally appropriate. Explain the procedure directly, honestly, and simply.
- Bring something distracting with you—anything your child likes to hold, listen to, or watch.
- Teach your child to help herself (Take an imaginary journey? Put on a "magic" sock?).
- Offer choices. Which arm? Sit up or lie down?

- Use a "hug hold" to provide emotional support for a blood draw. Hold the child on your lap. You hug the child, and the child hugs you. Let the health care staff do the rest.

For a biopsy, stronger medication is used to keep the child still and prevent pain. Stay close by and provide a familiar comfort item to help the child relax.[1]

Treatment

I feel mixed up about interferon. I'm going to have to do some serious investigating. What if the treatment could cause my daughter problems later in her life?

I sit here and think, "If I don't do it, this could happen. If I do it, this could happen." I make lists—and I pray a lot and ask for direction.

Patricia

I tried at first to keep it from him. I was devastated, and I needed time to think. Then I decided that at 10 years old he needs to be a part of this, to make decisions, just as I do about my treatment. I would never start treatment without his consent.

He can say, "I'm not ready. Can we think about this?" A positive attitude is powerful.

Irene

I put off my treatment so my daughter and I could do it together— so I could be a support to her. I did her shot, and she did mine. It helped both of us.

We'd lie in bed together and watch "Animal Planet." I'd notice that she would look pale and tired around her eyes. "Darn this hep C thing," she'd say.

"I know," I'd answer, "but we're doing the right thing."

Dana

Interferon Therapy. We have not yet defined the role of interferon therapy in treating children with hepatitis C. Many patients do not have symptoms, have normal or low ALT levels, and exhibit only mild liver injury and early stages of fibrosis on liver biopsy.

In addition, interferon therapy is difficult to maintain with young people. Complying with the strict regimen of shots and dealing with side effects present challenges. Interferon monotherapy (interferon alone) may be slightly more effective in children when compared to the adult experience, but rarely does this therapy lead to sustained viral clearance.

Despite these concerns, children with significant liver injury or fibrosis should be considered for treatment, even though the effects of this treatment on disease progression are unknown. Children should be referred to and evaluated by a pediatric gastroenterologist with experience in managing interferon therapy in this unique population.

Interferon Plus Ribavirin. Because the results of therapy with interferon monotherapy have been disappointing, researchers are currently conducting ongoing trials of the use of interferon alfa-2b plus ribavirin (combination therapy) in children with chronic hepatitis C in the United States. If combination therapy proves safe and effective, it may open the door to more successful future therapy for children with hepatitis C.

Pegylated Interferon. Researchers are just beginning to study the use of pegylated interferon for the treatment of chronic hepatitis C in children. No data is available to date.

Giving Injections. If a family chooses interferon therapy, it raises complex emotional issues. The parent must administer an injection and then deal with interferon's side effects. No parent likes to poke a child with needles. Often, the mother has gone through treatment herself and knows what side effects her child is facing.

"I do the first dose in the clinic," says Claassen, "and we watch the child for a couple of hours. I have the parents inject me with a saline solution so they get over the fear of entering someone's body with a needle. It's a sacred barrier."

Butler-Simon recommends that the parent allow the nurse to give her a saline injection so she can see how small the needle is and how much easier a subcutaneous (under the skin) injection is than an intramuscular one. "Am I inflicting pain: No. And the parent can see and feel that I'm not. That's what parents freak out about—hurting the child."

"Many parents have given a shot before—to themselves if they have hepatitis B or to a pet," says Claassen. "But still, even with experience, giving a shot to one's own child is different. We go through the steps to help them gain confidence, and they give the first shot here."

Tools that help parents, such as EMLA® Cream or ice to numb the skin, are like "training wheels," until the parent gains confidence. But it's a trade-off. The cream must stay on the skin for an hour, and during that hour anticipation and dread increase.

"First and foremost," says Butler-Simon, "is setting the attitude of the parent. Kids will respond to the parent's attitude, which should be 'no big deal, and if it is, we'll work through it,' rather than 'I'm so sorry, dear, but we have to do it.'"

Most parents want guidance on the mechanics of administering the injection. "For really young children, infants to age 3 or 4, it's best to give the shot in the butt," says Butler-Simon. "You can lay them in your lap with your leg over their legs, hanging them over your other leg, or place them on their belly on a couch. Distraction helps. Give them a doll that they can give a 'shot' to at the same time to help them feel that they have some control. Praise and stickers are helpful, but then move on. Don't drag the ritual out to the nth degree because you have to do it so frequently.

"At ages four to five, children may be able to be more cooperative. To elicit a sense of control, you can encourage them to do the alcohol swab, for example. For young school-age children, a 'hug-hold' is a good option. You hold the child on your lap. The child hugs you, you hug the child, and another adult gives the shot."

"Sometimes," says Claassen, "you have to come up with a good hold and get it over with. We've never had anyone fail therapy because it involves shots!"

Future Therapy. What if your child does not respond to interferon monotherapy or interferon plus ribavirin therapy? A number of new drugs and treatment strategies are in development or clinical trials. The trials of pegylated (long-acting) interferons plus ribavirin in adults are just undergoing review by the Food and Drug Administration (see Chapter 9). The future of treatment holds great hope for patients and families who are dealing with chronic hepatitis C.

Resources: For news of clinical trials for hepatitis C in children, contact PKIDs at 360-695-0293, website: www.pkids.org. Other websites that track clinical trials include www.centerwatch.com and the National Institutes of Health website: www.cc.nih.gov.

Resource: The American Liver Foundation created a national "Pediatric Liver Research Agenda 2000: A Blueprint for the Future, Research Goals and Strategies to Treat, Prevent, and Conquer Childhood Liver Diseases" under the leadership of Ronald Sokol, M.D., Director of Denver's Children's Hospital Pediatric General Clinical Research Center, Associate Medical Director of The Pediatric Liver Center, and Professor of Pediatrics at the University of Colorado Medical School. For a copy of the research agenda, call the ALF at 1-800-GO-LIVER, Ext. 136; website: www.liverfoundation.org/html/advores.htm.

Post-Treatment Follow-Up. Children who respond to interferon should be monitored for complete resolution of markers of viral infection. Non-responders to therapy should be monitored for disease progression.

Cirrhotic patients need to be monitored for early signs of liver decompensation (see Chapter 4). These patients are at greatest risk for development of liver cancer because they have both cirrhosis and active viral replication. Evidence of decompensation or development of isolated hepatoma (liver cancer) is an indication for referral for liver transplantation.

Despite these concerns and the need for monitoring, most children with chronic hepatitis C have a relatively benign course with few symptoms and slow progression of liver disease. Time is on their side as treatment options expand, and the likelihood of cure with medical therapy becomes increasingly possible.

A child is one who stands halfway
between an adult and a TV set.

Anonymous

Reference

1. Liver Center and Liver Transplantation Program of The Children's Hospital (Denver). "Preparing Children for Painful Procedures," Connections, Fall/Winter 2000, Vol. 13, No. 4: 4-5.

14

RESEARCH
TRENDS

Hope for the Future

In the years since my diagnosis in 1993, I've seen many advances in hepatitis C research: combination therapy, pegylated interferons, living-donor liver transplants. Even the once-held belief that cirrhosis is an irreversible death sentence is now being questioned by the HALT C trials.

With each revision of this book, we're able to move more topics from the research chapter to the treatment chapters as theories become reality. These exciting developments replace despair with hope. The future looks promising if we continue to raise public awareness and demand more research dollars.

Here's where we can do something. Each of us can talk about hepatitis C and educate others about this viral epidemic. Each of us can contribute time and money to finding the cure.

It's scary to know that a virus is circulating in your body, and that you can't get rid of it. Interferon-based therapies work for some people, but not for everyone. All of us who have been affected by hepatitis C know that there's got to be something better coming down the pike. And we wait and hope.

Hedy

As a hepatologist dealing with hepatitis C, I have observed great improvements in the treatment of this disease. However, even with the best antiviral regimen, nearly half of hepatitis C patients in the United States fail to respond. Nonetheless, antiviral research is blossoming, I look forward to the next few years, and I expect to see exciting new advances.

Hepatitis C research falls into two broad and somewhat overlapping categories: clinical research and basic research. Clinical research primarily determines whether new drug therapies are effective in treating hepatitis C. Basic research encompasses a wide variety of studies of hepatitis C, including, but not limited to: molecular biology, cell biology, cryobiology and liver cell transplantation, pathophysiology, and pharmacology.

In this final chapter, we'll cover the following topics:

- Clinical Research: Testing New Drugs
  Phases of Clinical Trials
  Should You Sign Up for a Study?
- Current Clinical Research for Treatment of Hepatitis C
  Thymosin
  New Interferon-Based Combinations
  IL-10
  Gamma-Interferon
  HALT C: Maintenance Therapy for Nonresponders with Fibrosis
  African Americans
- Potential New Therapies
  Vaccine Development
  Protease and Helicase Inhibitors
  Ribozymes
  Gene Therapy
- Basic Research
  Mechanisms of Resistance to Antiviral Therapy
  Animal and Cell Culture Models
  Mathematical Models
  Molecular Virology
  Cell Biology
  Cryobiology and Liver Cell Transplantation
  Pathophysiology
  Pharmacology

The Bioartificial Liver
• Research Funding

Clinical Research: Testing New Drugs

In the United States, pharmaceutical companies, the National Institutes of Health, and some large universities test promising new drugs and submit their results to the Food and Drug Administration (FDA). It is the responsibility of the FDA to critically examine the results of the studies and determine whether the new treatment is safe and effective through a careful system of checks and balances. State review boards also monitor studies and adverse reactions to medications. Drugs approved by the FDA become available to practicing physicians to use in the treatment of hepatitis C.

A well-defined process evaluates all new drugs. First, the drug's safety must be established through animal testing. These studies may also help to define the expected effectiveness and dose ranges of the drug when it is used later in humans. After a drug has undergone animal testing and has been approved by the FDA for clinical research with humans, the drug testing enters three phases.

Phases of Clinical Trials. Studies in Phase I (human toxicity) typically involve small numbers of patients or healthy controls who are given single doses of the drug in varying amounts. Patients are monitored very closely (physical examinations and blood testing) to detect any adverse effect of the medication. Researchers examine the absorption of the drug, its distribution in the body, metabolism, and elimination. Sometimes the cumulative toxicity of multiple doses of drug are examined in Phase I studies.

Phase II (dose finding) studies evaluate the response of the disease to the drug in large numbers of study subjects. Researchers determine the effectiveness of several different doses of the drug administered over prolonged periods of time to find the "optimal dose" for use in humans. Patients are also carefully monitored for evidence of toxicity.

Phase III (pre-clinical testing) typically treats hundreds to thousands of patients. Again, effectiveness and toxicity are carefully evaluated. Researchers often compare the drug under investigation to existing therapies and medications to obtain a measure of whether the new treatment represents an advance above current treatment strategies. These are the final studies done to obtain FDA approval and will determine how the drug is labeled. After this phase is completed, the results are submitted to the FDA for review. Although some drugs, such as those to treat cancer, AIDS, and ALS, are on a fast track for FDA approval, it may take approximately two years for other drugs to be approved. The FDA may approve the drug, reject it, or request more studies.

Ongoing clinical testing (post-marketing surveillance for problems that might arise) occurs after the FDA has approved the drug, usually for the first one to two years, and determines optimal ways to use the drug or new indications for using the drug.

Should You Sign Up for a Study? Obviously, before you enroll in a specific study, you should take time to review the patient informed consent document that you will have to sign. Be sure to ask how often you will see a doctor; doctor appointments vary at different study sites. You should also consider all the pros and cons of any study.

On the positive side:

1. You may get to try a new treatment that is not available through general clinical practice.
2. Typically, you would receive frequent examinations and careful follow-up.
3. Study coordinators will keep you informed about your status and progress.
4. Most studies are sponsored by either pharmaceutical companies or research grants, and typically your treatment is delivered without expense to you or your insurer. However, the degree of compensation can vary and you (or your insurer) may be responsible for some of the bill. Some studies also give extra compensation to you for expenses related to travel to the study site or for the time you spent participating in the research.
5. Your participation is kept confidential. Representatives from the FDA or study sponsors, however, have the right to review your study record.
6. You reserve the right to stop treatment and withdraw from the study at any time.

On the negative side:

1. Testing programs are rigid. You must make the time commitment to follow the protocol exactly. For example, you'll have to show up at certain times for follow-up tests.

2. Clinical trials are usually blinded. That means that you won't know what you're getting in terms of dosage or placebo, for example. If you have been given a placebo, the pharmaceutical company may offer the active drug to you (free of charge) at the end of your participation in the trial if you completed the study.
3. Sponsors can stop the trials at any time.
4. You may experience undocumented side effects.
5. You must be prepared to reveal all aspects of your physical and emotional health.
6. You won't know the results of the whole study, or your individual results, until every participant has completed the protocol. It may take more than a year from your point of enrollment.

If you fail to meet criteria for entry into the controlled studies, it is still possible to be treated with investigational drugs through compassionate-use protocols. Typically, drugs available on a compassionate-use basis have demonstrated effectiveness in studies but "registration trials" have not been done or completed and the drug has not received formal FDA approval. Physicians gain access to these drugs by contacting the pharmaceutical sponsor.

Current Clinical Research for Treatment of Hepatitis C

Optimum therapy for hepatitis C is under constant evaluation and reappraisal. One of the most exciting—and frustrating—parts of writing about clinical research is that by the time you read this chapter, researchers will be studying new treatments. As of August 2001, the following drugs were under investigation.

Thymosin. Thymosin, used alone, is ineffective in eradicating hepatitis C. One trial compared the effectiveness of the combination of thymosin plus interferon against interferon alone. The combination had more potent antiviral activity than interferon alone, because patients treated with the combination had lower levels of hepatitis C virus in their blood during treatment. In addition, more of the patients on combination therapy had a complete response (normal ALT) at end of treatment. However, relapse rates were high in both groups during a six-month period of post-treatment follow-up. Sustained response rates were only 6 percent. Current trials are examining the efficacy of pegylated interferon plus thymosin, but results of these studies have not yet been published.

New Interferon-Based Combinations. The search continues for alternatives to ribavirin to be used in combination with interferon to reduce the side effects and adverse reactions. A new form of ribavirin (L-ribavirin) does not cause hemolytic anemia and is currently undergoing investigation. Amantadine, which has few side effects, has been studied in several small trials with mixed results. Some investigators have examined triple therapy with interferon, ribavirin, and amantadine and suggest this regimen may be useful in treating nonresponders. Histamine analogues also show some synergism with interferon in the treatment of hepatitis C, but the magnitude of the response appears to be lower than that observed with ribavirin. Additional trials with histamine analogues are in process or planned.

The newest agent to be examined in combination protocols is mycophenolate mofetil. This compound is an immunosuppressant and is used in transplant recipients to prevent allograft rejection. However, the drug inhibits a specific lymphocyte enzyme, IMPDH (inosine monophosphate dehydrogenase), which is also a target of ribavirin. In addition, there has been some evidence from transplant studies that liver enzymes may be lower in transplant recipients with hepatitis C who are treated with mycophenolate mofetil. For this reason, some small studies have begun to examine the effectiveness of the combination of interferon with mycophenolate mofetil, and early results suggest that response may be similar to the combination of interferon plus ribavirin. However, mycophenolate mofetil is an immunosuppressant, and long-term use could theoretically potentially increase risk of infection and cancer. It suppresses the bone marrow production of white blood cells and can cause gastrointestinal distress. Additional trials are needed before any of the above combinations can reach clinical practice.

IL-10. Interleukin-10 (IL-10) has been evaluated mainly for its potential use as an anti-fibrotic agent. It is a naturally occurring compound in our bodies that regulates inflammatory reactions to infection or injury. Studies of model systems suggested that IL-10 could suppress inflammation and limit or even reverse fibrosis. One pilot study of a small number of patients with hepatitis C suggested that IL-10 could potentially reverse fibrosis.

For this reason, IL-10 was recently examined in a large multi-center trial where biopsies were performed at the start and periodically throughout the trial. Treatment biopsies demonstrated reduction in inflammation but no consistent improvement in fibrosis. In addition, side effects included headaches and dizziness, and there has been concern over possible neurotoxicity. The future of IL-10 in the treatment of hepatitis C remains uncertain.

Gamma-Interferon. Gamma-interferon is another potential anti-fibrotic agent, and, like IL-10, is a natural compound in our bodies that regulates inflammatory reactions to infection or injury. The group of hepatitis C patients targeted for this treatment is that of nonresponders to prior treatment with the combination of interferon-alfa plus ribavirin who have significant liver fibrosis. This group is at risk for clinical deterioration, need for liver transplantation, and development of liver cancer as the liver fibrosis progresses. The rationale for treatment is that inhibition or regression of fibrosis by gamma-interferon might reduce these risks. Trials of gamma-interferon in patients with chronic hepatitis C are currently being planned.

HALT C: Maintenance Therapy for Nonresponders with Fibrosis. The National Institutes of Health (NIH) has funded an eight-year multi-center trial to examine the ability of maintenance therapy with PEGASYS® (Roche) to reduce the rate of progression of liver fibrosis to cirrhosis and prevent clinical deterioration and liver cancer. Potential candidates for HALT C must be nonresponders to prior antiviral therapy (HCV-RNA positive throughout treatment) with significant amounts of fibrosis on liver biopsy. A number of ancillary studies will be conducted during this trial to examine several key virological, immunological, and clinical issues. Ten U.S. clinical centers are conducting HALT C.

Resource: For more information about HALT C, visit the NIH website at www.nih.gov or contact the NIH clinical center's patient recruitment and public liason office at 1-800-411-1212, (TTY: 1-866-411-1010).

African Americans. African Americans currently represent 12 to 13 percent of the U.S. population but account for approximately 22 percent of the 2.7 million U.S. citizens chronically infected with hepatitis C. Once infected, African Americans may be more susceptible to chronic infection, and genotype 1 appears to be more common. Despite the higher chance of developing chronic infection, African Americans seem to exhibit slower rates of progression to cirrhosis and advanced liver disease and less ability to clear hepatitis C with antiviral therapy.

Numerous potential explanations have been advanced to explain these racial differences in response to infection with hepatitis C. In response to this research need, the National Institute of Diabetes and Digestive and Kidney Diseases, National Cancer Institute, National Institute on Drug Abuse, National Institute of Allergy and Infectious Diseases, and the Office for Research on Minority Health convened a conference on December 2, 1999, entitled "Hepatitis C in African Americans." A number of key issues regarding hepatitis C infection in African Americans were highlighted and published (see Selected Bibliography at the back of this book). In addition, the NIH recently funded a multi-center study, VIRACEPT, to examine therapy and key aspects of hepatitis C infection in African Americans

Resource: Access the NIH website: www.nih.gov, VIRACEPT study, for more information.

Potential New Therapies

Vaccine Development. To date, researchers have made only partial and slow progress toward the development of a vaccine against hepatitis C. When vaccines were developed for hepatitis B, researchers knew that antibodies against a specific hepatitis B antigen protected against subsequent infection with hepatitis B.

Unfortunately, no naturally occurring protective antibodies have been identified for hepatitis C; all of the antibodies that have been identified do not protect against subsequent infection with hepatitis C. In addition, hepatitis C is genetically diverse, which makes it difficult to develop a single vaccine effective against all forms of the virus. Nonetheless, some advances have been made, and work is in progress.

Protease and Helicase Inhibitors. Recently, key viral enzymes have been identified, isolated, and crystallized: HCV proteases and helicase. HCV proteases are responsible for converting the large HCV protein into smaller proteins that are necessary for formation of viral particles. Proteases and helicase are essential for hepatitis C to complete its life cycle. For this reason, drugs or chemicals that inactivate HCV proteases and helicase would markedly inhibit viral assembly and secretion. At the time of this writing, a number of pharmaceutical firms are using the crystallographic data to design specific inhibitors.

Ribozymes. Ribozymes are RNA molecules that bind to specific regions of other RNAs and cleave the bound RNA (RNA RNAases). Recently, ribozymes have been synthesized that specifically bind to hepatitis C RNA and cleave the virus, inactivating it and preventing its replication. Phase I trials of the hepatitis C-specific ribozyme (Heptazyme™) have been completed with no adverse reactions noted. Phase II–III trials are just beginning as of August 2001.

Gene Therapy. As we learn more about the processes involved with viral replication and hepatocyte infection (cell biology), we may be able to construct biologic systems for clearing the virus from the cell. An example of this novel approach was recently published by Wu and colleagues.

These investigators were able to introduce a gene into cultured liver cells that produced an RNA that specifically inactivated hepatitis C. This RNA attached to a region in the hepatitis genes responsible for producing viral proteins. As a result, the production of viral proteins was markedly inhibited and viral replication ceased.

Obviously, this form of therapy is several years from clinical application. However, these early results suggest that gene therapy may be on the horizon as a potentially effective approach for hepatitis C.

Basic Research

Mechanisms of Resistance to Antiviral Therapy. This is a very important and emerging area of current and future research. Mechanisms of action of antiviral agents are currently under intense investigation. The converse, mechanisms of resistance to antiviral therapy, is now emerging as a related field of study.

Although the field is in its infancy, a number of observations are of interest and potentially important not only to hepatitis C but to viral infections in general. One intracellular system is of particular interest: oligoadenylate synthetase (2,5 OAS), RNAase L, and PKR. Future studies of this system may allow partial dissection of mechanisms of action of antivirals and potential means by which a virus resists clearance.

A related area of investigation is to examine mechanisms, virological and immunological, that occur with either clearance or chronic infection after acute hepatitis C in patients. This research is hampered by the inability to identify and study large groups of patients with early stages of acute infection.

Animal and Cell Culture Models. Studies of hepatitis C have been hampered by lack of a convenient experimental model of the infection. The ideal model for studying hepatitis C would be one that mimics the infection in humans and is affordable, widely available, and allows for easily reproducible manipulation of experimental conditions.

The chimpanzee is 98.5 percent genetically similar to humans and has served as the only animal model for this infection. A wide array of information has been gained from the study of hepatitis C in chimpanzees: viral transmission, time course of viral infection, characterization of the virus, and testing of infectivity of HCV clones. However, studies of hepatitis C in chimpanzees is difficult due to lack of availability and expense. The chimpanzee is the only primate susceptible to infection with hepatitis C. Other primates, including cynomolgus monkey, rhesus monkey, green monkey, Japanese monkey, and doguera baboon, have been intravenously inoculated with hepatitis C and failed to develop infection.

Results have been conflicting in transmission studies done with marmosets, tupaias, and tamarins. In addition, non-primates are not susceptible to infection with hepatitis C. It is of interest that the genes of small animals, such as the mouse, are very similar to their human counterparts, and studies are underway to develop genetically modified mice (transgenic) or mice maintaining human or chimpanzee liver cells (through a process called xenografting) that could sustain infection with hepatitis C.

Scientists have had limited success in developing of cell culture systems that express and maintain HCV replication. A number of cells have been examined, including hepatoma cell lines, transformed B-cells, transformed T-cells, primary liver cells, and isolated monocytes from circulating blood.

Recently, a part of the genome of hepatitis C has been demonstrated to continuously replicate in a human hepatoma cell line. Research to amplify this system to include the whole genome of hepatitis C is currently underway. Once this is achieved, investigators will be able to rapidly screen and examine effects of potential antiviral agents on replication of hepatitis C. However, these cell culture systems will still be inadequate for examining all aspects of hepatitis C infection and will give little or no information regarding mechanisms of progression of liver damage.

Mathematical Models. Recently, mathematical modeling has been used to measure kinetics of viral clearance in response to various treatments. This approach yields information concerning the rates of clearance of hepatitis C in response to antiviral regimens and may be useful in the early prediction of sustained virologic response. In addition, information is gained regarding the impact of age, gender, weight, race, and alcohol intake on the response to treatment.

One study used linear regression and prediction interval lines to compare HCV-RNA responses to four weeks of daily injections of standard interferon or combinations of 3 MU, 5 MU, or 10 MU plus ribavirin 1.0 to 1.2 g/d. Mathematical modeling determined that the estimated time to HCV-RNA negativity was greater than 12 weeks for standard interferon, 42 to 84 days for the 3 MU combination, 39 to 60 days for the 5 MU combination, and 25 to 45 days for the 10 MU combination. The authors of the study concluded that mathematical modeling might be useful in predicting differences in response between treatments from the characteristics of the early clearance of HCV-RNA. In other words, it might be possible to determine which of two treatments is likely to be most effective by conducting shorter term trials examining the early rate of viral clearance.

Mathematical modeling has also been used to probe potential mechanisms of action of antiviral regimens. The rate of decline in HCV-RNA during treatment with either pegylated or standard interferon was examined in 33 patients with chronic hepatitis C. The investigators correlated sustained virologic clearance with a "second-phase" clearance of HCV-RNA. The latter clearance is thought to represent the rate of degradation of infected cells. The data suggested that one mechanism of the improved efficacy of pegylated interferon could be enhancement of the rate of death of infected cells. Differences in response were noted between the various genotypes of HCV.

Molecular Virology. Researchers have made amazing advances in understanding the hepatitis C virus, in large part because of techniques available through the new scientific field of molecular biology. As a result, scientists have completely defined the genetic makeup of the hepatitis C virus. Despite these advances, however, we still lack basic information about the proteins produced by this virus and how these proteins interact with one another and with the host cell.

Current studies are evaluating the types and properties of the proteins produced by the hepatitis C genes. It is likely that these studies will unlock the mechanisms of viral protein assembly, viral formation, and secretion of the virus out of the liver cell into blood. Understanding these critical steps required to maintain the hepatitis C infection will allow scientists to develop medications or strategies to stop the virus from reproducing (replicating) and, ultimately, to eradicate the infection.

Additional studies are trying to define how the hepatitis C virus genes control and regulate the virus's production of proteins and allow the virus to copy its own genes to make new virus. Replication maintains the infection; without it, hepatitis C would disappear after a period of time. Scientists, therefore, are looking for keys to designing drugs that will stop viral replication.

One current area of development is HCV-specific proteases and helicase inhibitors, discussed earlier. As of this writing, none are in clinical trials. However, protease inhibitors are under development, and we anticipate that many will be tested in humans in the next few years. These inhibitors will inactivate the enzymes necessary for creating the molecules that form viral particles that are secreted from the liver cell and then reinfect adjacent cells. It is likely that inhibitors and other "designer" drugs will have a major impact on the treatment of hepatitis C.

Cell Biology. Despite what we do know about the hepatitis C genes and many of the proteins produced, little is known about the interaction between the hepatitis C virus and the liver cell. Future studies in this area should yield fruitful information for designing therapies, but right now many questions remain unanswered, including the following:

- What attracts hepatitis C to the liver and not to other tissues?
- How does hepatitis C bind to the surface of a liver cell and get into it?
- Once hepatitis C enters the liver cell, how does it survive?
- Why doesn't the liver cell simply swallow it up and digest it?
- What cellular systems in the liver cell are required to aid the replication of the virus?
- What are the key determinants of assembly of the viral proteins and genes to form an active infectious particle?
- What processes within the liver cell control the secretion of the viral particle out of the cell?

Cryobiology and Liver Cell Transplantation. An emerging field that is extremely exciting for both research applications and potential therapies is the isolation, storage, and subsequent use of human liver cells. These techniques have only recently become available with the development of human liver cell banks.

It's possible to freeze and store (cryopreserve) human liver cells taken from several specimens of human livers recovered for use in organ transplantation but rejected due to fatty change or physical damage to the organ. After sterile preparation, cells may be stored in a specialized cryopreservation medium for later thawing and use. Thawed cells are subsequently infused into patients with acute fulminant liver failure. In some cases, this technique has been successful at reversing some of the complications of liver failure and temporarily sustaining life.

Despite these initial promising results, in no case has liver cell transplantation saved patients independent of liver transplantation. Nonetheless, human liver cells have many major potential useful research applications, especially for studying the molecular virology and cell biology of hepatitis C. It is anticipated that researchers will be able to define the entire life cycle of hepatitis C with appropriate experiments using these cells.

Pathophysiology. One interesting feature of hepatitis C (and viral hepatitis in general) is that the hepatitis C infection probably is not sufficient to destroy or damage liver cells by itself. We don't fully understand the complex process of liver cell injury and the formation of fibrous tissue in the liver. Finally, repair mechanisms, such as liver regeneration, are poorly defined.

Many different laboratories are studying the effects of cofactors that may contribute to liver cell injury, fibrosis, regeneration, and progression to cirrhosis. These cofactors include processes such as excessive iron accumulation, oxidative stress, abnormal bile salts, and inflammatory mediators released by immune cells.

In the absence of effective therapies to eradicate hepatitis C, therapies that can modify basic mechanisms of cell injury and fibrosis may reduce the rate of progression to cirrhosis and the need for liver transplantation, slow the progression to liver failure, and reduce the rate of death from liver disease.

Pharmacology. As you can see, it's easy to understand that future treatment of hepatitis C could involve medications that target many different sites. I've briefly mentioned proteases and helicase inhibitors, which directly target the virus. Antiviral agents that interfere with the assembly or secretions of viral genes or proteins may soon be developed.

In the absence of effective antiviral agents, treatments could focus on the mechanisms of liver cell injury. Antioxidants might be used to reduce the risk of oxidative liver cell injury. Iron removal by phlebotomy (drawing blood) may reduce storage of iron within the liver, perhaps reducing liver cell injury. Specific drugs may be developed to inhibit liver fibrosis. Undoubtedly, numerous other points of attack will be defined as our knowledge expands in the fields of molecular virology, cell biology, and pathophysiology of chronic hepatitis C.

The Bioartificial Liver. Patients who suffer from chronic kidney failure have an option, short of transplantation, that prolongs life: dialysis. Unfortunately, patients with chronic liver disease do not have a comparable liver dialysis machine.

. Recently, several laboratories have begun to examine the effectiveness of bioartificial livers. Like dialysis machines, the patient's blood is passed through a capillary system to filter and cleanse the blood. The difference between standard dialysis and bioartificial livers is that liver cells are inserted into the capillary system.

The liver cells may be necessary to make the system function more like a normal liver. Theoretically, these functioning liver cells should help detoxify the patient's blood. In addition, researchers have suggested that substances synthesized and secreted by the liver cells may gain entry back into the blood and further support the patient.

Conceptually, many of the aspects of the bioartificial liver machine are sound and make sense. On the other hand, many technical problems limit the success of these machines. In the first place, the liver cells survive for only a short period of time, and cartridges need to be replaced frequently. Second, the cost of performing the dialysis is excessive. Third, the capillary barrier between plasma and liver cells is great and does not duplicate the processes of exchange between normal blood and liver cells in the patient. As of this writing, bioartificial liver machines are still considered highly experimental.

Research Funding

It is my hope that we are entering a new era in the treatment of hepatitis C, where research may ultimately lead to discoveries of more effective treatments that benefit patients. Research into the basic mechanisms of hepatitis C replication and infection of the liver cell is absolutely essential, so that our understanding and treatment of this devastating disease may leap forward.

Funds for hepatitis C research at the National Institutes of Health increased from $39.7 million in 1999 to an estimated $49 million in fiscal year 2000. In addition, the National Institute of Diabetes and Digestive and Kidney Diseases, the National Institute of Allergy and Infectious Diseases, and other NIH centers awarded 29 HCV research grants. [1]

This is a step in the right direction, but it's obvious that we do not yet understand the enormous financial—let alone emotional—scope of the HCV crisis. A recent report issued by Milliman & Robertson, Inc., developed an actuarial model to evaluate the economic impact of hepatitis C on the U.S. population. It found that people with HCV currently consume at least $15 billion per year for all their medical care. Without effective curative treatment (defined in the report as combination therapy, interferon-alfa plus ribavirin) total health care costs for patients infected with hepatitis C will peak at an estimated $26 billion (in current dollars) per year in about 2021."[2]

Clearly, research that results in better treatment ultimately saves money as well as lives. Hepatitis C patients, friends, and family members must focus attention on research. We must make it our top priority to confront, define, and eradicate this serious viral infection, chronic hepatitis C.

Where observation is concerned,
chance favors only the prepared mind.

Louis Pasteur

References

1. Hepatitis Foundation International. "Walk on Washington—Mission Accomplished," Hepatitis Alert, Summer 2000:1.
2. Dulworth, Sherrie, RN, Sunit Patel, FSA, MAAA, Bruce S. Pyenson, FSA, MAAA. "The Hepatitis Epidemic: Looking at the Tip of the Iceberg," Milliman & Robertson, Inc. 2000:1.

Resources

Organizations

American Liver Foundation (ALF)
75 Maiden Lane, Suite 603
New York, NY 10038-4810
1-800-GO-LIVER
1-888-4-HEP-ABC
1-888-4-HEP-USA
Website: www.liverfoundation.org
Email: www.webmail@liverfoundation.org

The Hep C Connection
1177 Grant Street
Suite 200
Denver, CO 80203
303-860-0800
HepC Hotline: 1-800-522-HEPC
Website: www.hepc-connection.org
Email: info@hepc-connection.org

Hepatitis C Awareness Project
P.O. Box 41803
Eugene, OR 97404
541-607-5725
Email: hepcaware@aol.com

Hepatitis C Global Foundation
1404 Madison Avenue
Redwood City, CA 94061
650-369-0330
Website: www.hepcglobal.org
Email: jtranchina@hepcglobal.org

Hepatitis C Prison Coalition
P.O. Box 41803
Eugene, OR 97404
541-607-5725
Website: www.hcvprisonnews.org
Email: hepcaware@aol.com

Hepatitis C Support Project
P.O. Box 427037
San Francisco, CA 94142
415-978-2400
Website: www.hcvadvocate.org
Email: sfhepcat@pacbell.net

Hepatitis Education Project
4603 Aurora Avenue North
Seattle, WA 98103-6513
1-800-218-6932
206-732-0311
Website: www.scn.org/health/hepatitis/index.htm
Email: hep@scn.org

Hepatitis Foundation International (HFI)
30 Sunrise Terrace
Cedar Grove, NJ 07009-1423
1-800-891-0707
Website: www.hepfi.org
Email: HFI@intac.com

Latino Organization for Liver Awareness (LOLA)
P.O. Box 842, Throggs Neck Station
Bronx, NY 10465
1-888-367-LOLA
Website: www.lola-national.org
Email: mdlola@aol.com

National Hepatitis C Advocacy Council (NHCAC)
Website: www.hepcnetwork.org

Parents of Kids with Infectious Diseases (PKIDs)
P.O. Box 5666
Vancouver, WA 98668
1-877-55-PKIDS
360-695-0293
Website: www.pkids.org
Email: pkids@pkids.org

Veterans Aimed Towards Awareness
111 West Main Street
Middletown, DE 19709
302-633-5357
Website: www.veteranshepaware.com
Email: bakfield@aol.com

Government Agencies

Centers for Disease Control and Prevention (CDC)
Hepatitis Branch, Mailstop G37
1600 Clifton Road N.E.
Atlanta, GA 30333
404-639-3311
CDC Hepatitis Hotline: 1-888-443-7232
CDC Public Inquiries: 1-800-311-3435
Website: http: www.cdc.gov/ncidod/diseases/hepatitis/
Email: dvd1hep@cdc.gov

Departments of Public Health
For information about hepatitis C in your state, call your State Department of Public Health, Epidemiology Division.

The National Institutes of Health (NIH) is the largest biomedical research center in the world. It's the research arm of the Public Health Service, U.S. Department of Health and Human Services; 301-496-1776 (Visitor Information Center); Website: www.nih.gov. A helpful resource is CHID Online (Combined Health Information Database); Website: www.chid.nih.gov.

Among its institutes that conduct and support research on hepatitis viruses are the National Institute of Allergy and Infectious Diseases (NIAID) and the National Institute of Diabetes & Digestive & Kidney Diseases (NIDDK):

National Institute of Allergy and Infectious Diseases (NIAID)
The NIAID has the largest budget for research into viral hepatitis. For an informational packet on hepatitis C, write to:
NIAID Office of Communications
Building 31
Room 7A50
Bethesda, MD 20892
301-496-5717
Press releases, fact sheets, and other materials are available on the Internet via the NIAID home page: www.niaid.nih.gov.

National Institute of Diabetes & Digestive & Kidney Diseases (NIDDK)
For a packet of materials on hepatitis C, write to:
National Digestive Diseases Information Clearinghouse (NDDIC)
2 Information Way
Bethesda, MD 20892-3570
Website: www.niddk.nih.gov
Email: nddic@info.niddk.nih.gov

Transplant Organizations and Agencies

Children's Liver Alliance
3835 Richmond Avenue
Box 190
Staten Island, NY 10312
718-987-6200
Website: http://livertx.org
Email: livers4kids@earthlink.net

Transplant Recipient International Organization (TRIO)
Nationwide support group for patients and families
1000 16th Street N.W.
Suite 602
Washington, DC 20036-5705
1-800-TRIO-386
202-293-0980
Website: www.trioweb.org

United Network for Organ Sharing (UNOS)
1100 Boulders Parkway
Suite 500
P.O. Box 13770
Richmond, VA 23225-8770
804-330-8500
Patient information: 1-888-TX INFO1 (1-888-894-6361)
Website: www.unos.org

U.S. Department of Health and Human Services
Division of Transplantation
5600 Fishers Lane
Room 481
Rockville, MD 20857
301-443-7577
Website: www.hrsa.gov/osp/dot
Website: www.organdonor.gov

Note: Multiple Internet sites with information on hepatitis C exist. Although many have important information, we do not specifically endorse any of these sites although we have used resources from government-based websites in the production of this book.

Selected Bibliography

Chapter 1

Alter, H.J., R.H. Purcell, J.W. Shih, J.C. Melpolder, M. Houghton, Q.L. Choo, G. Kou. 1989. Detection of Antibody to Hepatitis C Virus in Prospectively Followed Transfusion Recipients with Acute and Chronic Non-A, Non-B Hepatitis. *New England Journal of Medicine.* 321:1494-1500.

Alter, M.J., H.S. Margolis, K. Krawczynski, F.N. Judson, A. Mares, W.J. Alexander, P.Y. Hu, J.K. Miller, M.A. Gerber, R.E. Sampliner, E.L. Meeks, M.J. Beach. 1992. The Natural History of Community-Acquired Hepatitis C in the United States. *New England Journal of Medicine.* 327:1899-905.

Everson, G.T. 2001. "Natural History of Hepatitis C." *Chronic Viral Hepatitis: Diagnosis and Management.* R.S. Koff, G.Y. Wu, eds. Totowa: Humana Press. (160 refs)

"Global Prevalence of Hepatitis C." 1999. *World Health Organization.* http://www/who.int/emc/images/hepacmap.jpg. 17 May 2001.

Kou, G., Q.L. Choo, H.J. Alter, G.L. Gitnick, A.G. Redeker, R.H. Purcell, T. Miyamura, J.L. Dienstag, M.J. Alter, C.E. Stevens, G.E. Tegtmeier, F. Bonino, M. Colombo, W.S. Lee, C. Kou, K. Berger, J.R. Shuster, L.R. Overby, D.W. Bradley, M. Houghton. 1989. An Assay for Circulating Antibodies to a Major Etiologic Virus of Human Non-A, Non-B Hepatitis. *Science.* 244:362-364.

Mandell, G.L., J.E. Bennett, R. Dolin, eds. 1995. *Principles and Practice of Infectious Diseases,* Vol.2. New York: Churchill Livingstone.

National Institutes of Health. 1997. *Management of Hepatitis C.* NIH Consensus Statement 1997. Mar 24-26; 15(3):1-41.

Radetsky, P. 1994. *The Invisible Invaders: Viruses and the Scientists Who Pursue Them*. Boston: Little, Brown and Co.

"Viral Hepatitis C Fact Sheet." 16 April 2001. *National Center for Infectious Diseases. Centers for Disease Control and Prevention*. http://www.cdc.gov/ncidod/diseases/hepatitis/c/fact.htm. 11 May 2001.

"Hepatitis C/Fact Sheet No. 164." Oct. 2000. *World Health Organization*. http://www.who.int/inf-fs/en/fact164.html. 17 May 2001.

Chapter 2

Bren, Linda. "Hepatitis C: An Update." Food and Drug Administration. *FDA Consumer*. July-Aug. 2001.Vol. 35. No. 4:24-29.

"FDA Approves First Home Test for Hepatitis C Virus. 29 April 1999. Food and Drug Administration. http://www.fda.gov/bbs/topics/ANSWERS/ANS00952.html. 1 June 2001.

Kato, N., O.Yokosuka, M. Omata, K. Hosoda, M. Ohto. 1990. Detection of Hepatitis C Virus Ribonucleic Acid in the Serum by Amplification with Polymerase Chain Reaction. *Journal of Clinical Investigation*. 86:1764-1767.

Lau, J.Y.N., G.L. Davis, L.E. Prescott, G. Maertens, K.L. Lindsay, K.P. Qian, M. Mizokami, P. Simmonds, and Hepatitis Interventional Therapy Group. 1996. Distribution of Hepatitis C Virus Genotypes Determined by Line Probe Assay in Patients with Chronic Hepatitis C Seen at Tertiary Referral Centers in the United States. *Annals of Internal Medicine*. 124:868-76.

Ohno, T., J.Y.N. Lau. 1996. The "Gold-Standard," Accuracy, and the Current Concepts: Hepatitis C Virus Genotype and Viremia (editorial). *Hepatology*. 24:1312-1315.

Pawlotsky, J-M, M. Bouvier-Alias, C. Hezode, F. Darthuy, J. Remire, D. Dhumeaux. 2000. Standardization of Hepatitis C Virus RNA Quantitation. *Hepatology*. 32:654-659.

Saadeh, S., G. Cammell, W. D. Carey, Z.Younossi, D. Barnes, K. Easley. 2001. The Role of Liver Biopsy in Chronic Hepatitis C. *Hepatology*. 33:196-200.

Sarrazin, C., G. Teuber, R. Kokka, H. Rabenau, S. Zeuzem. 2000. Detection of Residual Hepatitis C Virus RNA by Transcription-Mediated Amplification in Patients with Complete Virologic Response According to Polymerase Chain Reaction-Based Assays. *Hepatology.* 32:818-823.

Zein, N.N., J. Rakela, E. Krawitt, K.R. Reddy, T. Tominaga, D. Persing, and the Collaborative Study Group. 1996. Hepatitis C Virus Genotypes in the United States: Epidemiology, Pathogenicity, and Response to Interferon Therapy. *Annals of Internal Medicine.* 125:634-640.

Chapter 3

Alter, H.J., C. Conry-Cantilena, J. Melpolder, D. Tan, M. Van Raden, D. Herion, D. Lau, J.H. Hoofnagle. 1997. Hepatitis C in Asymptomatic Blood Donors. *Hepatology:*26 (Suppl 1):29S-33S.

Alter, M.J., D. Kruszon-Moran, O.V. Nainan, G.M. McQuillan, F. Gao, L.A. Moyer, R.A. Kaslow, H.S. Margolis. 1999. The Prevalence of Hepatitis C Virus Infection in the United States, 1988 through 1994. *New England Journal of Medicine.* 341:556-562.

"Basic Guidelines for Getting a Tattoo." *Alliance of Professional Tattoists.* http://www..safetattoos.com/faq.htm. 30 May 2001.

Benamouzig, R., V. Ezratty, S. Chaussade. 1990. Risk for Type C Hepatitis Through Sexual Contact (editorial). *Annals of Internal Medicine.* 113:638.

Bourliere, M., P. Halfon, Y. Quentin, P. David, C. Mengotti, I. Portal, H. Khiri, S. Benali, H. Perrier, C. Boustiere, M. Jullien, G. Lambot. 2000. Covert Transmission of Hepatitis C Virus During Bloody Fisticuffs. *Gastroenterology.* 119:507-511.

Castrone, L. 2 July 1996. Piercing and Tattooing, Body Language of 90s Worries Health Experts. *Rocky Mountain News.* 3D.

Donahue, J.G., A. Munoz, P.M. Ness, D.E. Brown, D.H. Yawn, H.A. McAllister, B.A. Reitz, K.E. Nelson. 1992. The Declining Risk of Post-transfusion Hepatitis C Virus Infection. *New England Journal of Medicine.* 327:369-73.

Esteban, J.I., A. González, J.M. Hernández, L. Viladomiu, C. Sánchez, J.C. López-Talavera, D. Lucea, C. Martin-Vega, X. Vidal, R. Esteban, J. Guardia. 1990. Evaluation of Antibodies to Hepatitis C Virus in a Study of Transfusion-Associated Hepatitis. *New England Journal of Medicine.* 323:1107-1112.

Everhart, J.E., A.M. Di Bisceglie, L.M. Murray, H.J. Alter, J.J. Melpolder, G. Kuo, J. Hoofnagle. 1990. Risk for Non-A, Non-B (Type C) Hepatitis Through Sexual or Household Contact with Chronic Carriers. *Annals of Internal Medicine.* 112:544–545.

"Government Urges Safer Needles." Food and Drug Administration. *FDA Consumer.* March–April 2000:2.

Haley, R.W., R.P. Fischer. 2001. Commercial Tattooing as a Potentially Important Source of Hepatitis C Infection: Clinical Epidemiology of 626 Consecutive Patients Unaware of Their Hepatitis C Serologic Status. *Medicine.* 80:134–151.

Hollinger, F.B., J.L. Hsiang. 1992. Community-Acquired Hepatitis C Virus Infection (editorial). *Gastroenterology.* 102:1425–29.

Kelen, G.D., G.B. Green, R.H. Purcell, D.W. Chan, B.F. Qaqish, K.T. Sivertson, T.C. Quinn. 1992. Hepatitis B and Hepatitis C in Emergency Department Patients. *New England Journal of Medicine.* 326:1399–404.

Koff, R.S. 1992. The Low Efficiency of Maternal-Neonatal Transmission of Hepatitis C Virus: How Certain Are We? (editorial). *Annals of Internal Medicine.* 117:967–969.

Long, G.E., L.S. Rickman. 1994. Infectious Complications of Tattoos. *Clinical Infectious Diseases.* 18:610–9.

Mannucci, P.M., K. Schimpf, B. Brettler, N. Ciavarella, M. Colombo, F. Haschke, K. Lechner, J. Lusher, G. Weissbach, and the International Study Group. 1990. Low Risk for Hepatitis C in Hemophiliacs Given a High-Purity, Pasteurized Factor VIII Concentrate. *Annals of Internal Medicine.* 113:27–32.

McCashland, T.M., T.L. Wright, J.P. Donovan, D.F. Schafer, M.F. Sorrell, T.G. Heffron, A.N. Langnas, I.J. Fox, B.W. Shaw, Jr., R.K. Zetterman. 1995. Low Incidence of Intraspousal Transmission of Hepatitis C Virus after *Liver Transplantation. Liver Transplantation and Surgery.* 1:358–361.

Mitsui, T., K. Iwano, K. Masuko, C. Yamazaki, H. Okamoto, F. Tsuda, T. Tanaka, S. Mishiro. 1992. Hepatitis C Virus Infection in Medical Personnel After Needlestick Accident. *Hepatology.* 16:1109–1114.

"Needle Safety Jabs World's Attention." Hepatitis Foundation International. *Hepatitis Alert.* Summer 2000: 6.

Ohto, H., S. Terazawa, N. Sasaki, N. Sasaki, K. Hino, C. Ishiwata, M. Kako, N. Ujiie, C. Endo, A. Matsui, H. Okamoto, S. Mishiro, and the Vertical Transmission of Hepatitis C Virus Collaborative Study Group. 1994. Transmission of Hepatitis C Virus from Mothers to Infants. *New England Journal of Medicine.* 330:744-50.

Pereira, B.J.G., E.L. Milford, R.L. Kirkman, A.S. Levey. 1991. Transmission of Hepatitis C Virus by Organ Transplantation. New England Journal of Medicine. 325:454-60.

Pereira, B.J.G., E.L. Milford, R.L. Kirkman, S. Quan, K.R. Sayre, P.J. Johnson, J.C. Wilber, A.S. Levey. 1992. Prevalence of Hepatitis C Virus RNA in Organ Donors Positive for Hepatitis C Antibody and in the Recipients of Their Organs. *New England Journal of Medicine.* 327:910-5.

Roth, D., J.A. Fernandez, S. Babischkin, A. De Mattos, B.E. Buck, S. Quan, L. Olson, G.W. Burke, J.R. Nery, V. Esquenazi, E.R. Schiff, J. Miller. 1992. Detection of Hepatitis C Virus Infection among Cadaver Organ Donors: Evidence for Low Transmission of Disease. *Annals of Internal Medicine.* 117:470-475.

Roudot-Thoraval, F., J. Pawlotsky, V. Thiers, L. Deforges, P. Girollet, F. Guillot, C. Huraux, P. Aumont, C. Brechot, D. Dhumeaux. 1993. Lack of Mother-to-infant Transmission of Hepatitis C Virus in Human Immunodeficiency Virus-seronegative Women: A Prospective Study with Hepatitis C Virus RNA Testing. *Hepatology.* 17:772-777.

Rumi, M.G., M. Colombo, A. Gringeri, P.M. Mannucci. 1990. High Prevalence of Antibody to Hepatitis C Virus in Multitransfused Hemophiliacs with Normal Transaminase Levels. *Annals of Internal Medicine.* 112:379-380.

Schiff, E.R. 1992. Hepatitis C Among Health Care Providers: Risk Factors and Possible Prophylaxis (editorial). *Hepatology.* 16:1300-1301.

Schreiber, G.B., M.P. Busch, S.H. Kleinman, J.J. Korelitz, for the Retrovirus Epidemiology Donor Study. 1996. The Risk of Transfusion-Transmitted Viral Infections. *New England Journal of Medicine.* 334:1685-90.

Seeff, L.B., H.J. Alter. 1994. Spousal Transmission of the Hepatitis C Virus? (editorial). *Annals of Internal Medicine.* 120:807–809.

Seeff, L.B., Z. Buskell-Bales, E.C. Wright, S.J. Durako, H.J. Alter, F.L. Iber, F.B. Hollinger, G. Gitnick, R.G. Knodell, R.P. Perrillo, C.E. Stevens, C.G. Hollingsworth, and National Heart, Lung, and Blood Institute Study Group. 1992. Long-term Mortality after Transfusion-Associated Non-A, Non-B Hepatitis. *New England Journal of Medicine.* 327:1906–11.

Shakil, A.O., C. Conry-Cantilena, H.J. Alter, P. Hayashi, D.E. Kleiner, V. Tadeschi, K. Krawczynski, H.S. Conjeevaram, R. Sallie, A.M. Di Bisceglie, and Hepatitis C Study Group. 1995. Volunteer Blood Donors with Antibody to Hepatitis C Virus: Clinical, Biochemical, Virologic, and Histologic Features. *Annals of Internal Medicine.* 123:330–337.

"Summary of Findings from the 1999 National Household Survey on Drug Abuse." 10 Oct. 2000. *Substance Abuse and Mental Health Services Administration.*

Tong, M.J., N.S. El-Farra, A.R. Reikes, R.L. Co. 1995. Clinical Outcomes after Transfusion-Associated Hepatitis C. *New England Journal of Medicine.* 332:1463–6.

U.S. Department of Health and Human Services, Food and Drug Administration, Center for Biologics Evaluation and Research. March 1998. *Supplemental Testing and the Notification of Consignees of Donor Test Results for Antibody to Hepatitis C Virus (Anti-HCV).* Rockville: Office of Communication, Training and Manufacturers Assistance (HFM-40).

Chapter 4

Hamilton, E. 1940, reprint 1989. *Mythology, Timeless Tales of Gods and Heroes.* Reprint. New York: Meridian.

Lauer, G. M., B. C. Walker. 2001. Hepatitis C Virus Infection. *New England Journal of Medicine.* 345:41–52.

Lyons, A.S., J.R. Petrucelli, II. 1978. *Medicine, An Illustrated History.* New York: Harry N. Abrams.

Mehta, S. H., F. L. Brancati, M. S. Sulkowski, S. A. Strathdee, M. Szklo, D. L. Thomas. 2000. Prevalence of Type 2 Diabetes Mellitus among Persons with Hepatitis C Virus Infection in the United States. *Annals of Internal Medicine.* 133:592-599.

Neruda, Pablo. 1977. *Nuevas Odas Elementales, Cuarta Edicion.* Buenos Aires; Editorial Losada.

"Sculpture in Spain Salutes the 'Silent, Unselfish' Liver." *Austin American-Statesman.* 28 June 1987: A2.

Chapter 5

Angell, M., J.P. Kassirer. 1998. Alternative Medicine – The Risks of Untested and Unregulated Remedies. *New England Journal of Medicine.* 339:839-841.

Boigk, G., L. Stroedter, H. Herbst, J. Waldschmidt, E. O. Riecken, D. Schuppan. 1997. Silymarin Retards Collagen Accumulation in Early and Advanced Biliary Fibrosis Secondary to Complete Bile Duct Obliteration in Rats. *Hepatology.* 26:643-649.

Breidenbach, T.H., M.W. Hoffman, T.H. Becker, H. Schlitt, J. Klempnauer. 27 May 2000. Drug Interaction of St. John's Wort with Cyclosporine. *Lancet.* 355:1912.

Caregaro, L., F. Alberino, P. Amodio, C. Merkel, M. Bolognesi, P. Angeli, A. Gatta. 1996. Malnutrition in Alcoholic and Virus-Related Cirrhosis. *American Journal of Clinical Nutrition.* 63:602-9.

Coppes, M.J., R.A. Anderson, R.M. Egeler, J.E.A. Wolff. 1998. Alternative Therapies for the Treatment of Childhood Cancer. *New England Journal of Medicine.* 339:846.

Cowley, J., 1996. Herbal Warning. *Newsweek.* 6 May, 63.

DiPaola, R.S., H. Zhang, G.H. Lambert, R. Meeker, E. Licitra, M.M. Rafi, B.T. Zhu, H. Spaulding, S. Goodin, M.B. Toledano, W.N. Hait, M.A. Gallo. 1998. Clinical and Biologic Activity of an Estrogenic Herbal Combination (PC-SPES) in Prostate Cancer. *New England Journal of Medicine.* 339:785-791.

Eisenberg, D.M. 1997. Advising Patients Who Seek Alternative Medical Therapies. *Annals of Internal Medicine*. 127:61-69.

Greenwald, John. 1998. Herbal Healing. *Time*, 23 November, 60-69.

Gugliotta, Guy. "Supplements Aren't So Healthy." *Denver Post*. 19 March 2000: 5A.

Henkel, John. "fda.gov/A Look at Medical Alternatives." *FDA Consumer*. May-June 2001: 34.

Ko, R.J. 1998. Adulterants in Asian Patent Medicines. *New England Journal of Medicine*. 339:847.

Kurtzweil, Paula. 1998. An FDA Guide to Dietary Supplements. *FDA Consumer*. Vol.32 No.5:28-35.

Larrey, D., F. P. Pageaux. August 1995. Hepatotoxicity of Herbal Remedies and Mushrooms. *Seminars in Liver Disease*. 15:183-188.

Marquis, Christopher. 2000. "90% of U.S. Diets Lacking, Feds Say." *Denver Post*. 28 May, 24A.

"Medicines and Your Liver." Hepatitis Foundation International. *Hepatitis Alert*. Summer 2000. 5.

Munoz, S.J. 1991. Nutritional Therapies in Liver Disease. *Seminars in Liver Disease*. 11:278-291.

"NBJ's Fifth Annual Overview of the Nutrition Industry," *Nutrition Business Journal*. Vol.V No. 7/8 2000: 1, 3-7.

Nompleggi, D.J., H.L. Bonkovsky. 1994. Nutritional Supplementation in Chronic Liver Disease: An Analytical Review. *Hepatology*. 19:518-533.

"Q and A's on Dietary Guidelines for Americans, 2000." 3 June 2000. *Center for Nutrition Policy and Promotion*. 1 Sept. 2000. http://www.usda.gov/cnpp/Pubs/DG2000/Qa5-2.pdf.

"Research Funding Up for Alternative Medicine." Hepatitis Foundation International. *Hepatitis Alert*. Spring 2000, Vol.VI, No. 2: 6.

Schuppan, D., J.D. Jia, B. Brinkhaus, E.G. Hahn. 1999. Herbal Products for Liver Disease: A Therapeutic Challenge for the New Millennium. *Hepatology.* 30:1099-1104.

Slifman, N.R., W.R. Obermeyer, S.M. Musser, W.A. Correll, S.M. Cichowicz, J.M. Betz, L.A. Love. 1998. Contamination of Botanical Dietary Supplements by Digitalis Lanata. *New England Journal of Medicine.* 339:806-811.

U.S. Department of Agriculture, U.S. Department of Health and Human Services. 1995. *Dietary Guidelines for Americans.* Fourth Edition. Washington.

Woolf, G.M., L.M. Petrovic, S.E. Rojter, S. Wainwright, F.G. Villamil, W.N. Katkov, P. Michieletti, I.R. Wanless, F.R. Stermitz, J.J. Beck, J.M. Vierling. 1994. Acute Hepatitis Associated with the Chinese Herbal Product Jin Bu Huan. *Annals of Internal Medicine.* 121:729-735.

Chapter 6

Anderson, Greg. 1993. 50 *Essential Things to Do When the Doctor Says It's Cancer.* New York: Plume/Penguin.

Benson, Herbert with Marg Stark. 1996. *Timeless Healing, the Power and Biology of Belief.* New York: Scribner.

Benson, Herbert with Miriam Z. Klipper. 1975. *The Relaxation Response.* New York: Avon.

LeShan, Lawrence. 1994. *Cancer As a Turning Point.* New York. Plume/Penguin.

Moyers, Bill. 1993. *Healing and the Mind.* New York/Doubleday.

Spiegel, David, M.D. 1993. *Living Beyond Limits.* New York: Random House.

Topf, Linda Noble with Hal Z. Bennett. 1995. *You Are Not Your Illness.* New York: Fireside.

Chapter 7

Beam, Jr., Burton T. and Kenn B. Tacchino. Jan. 1997. *The Health Insurance Portability and Accountability Act of 1996.* Journal of the American Society of CLU & ChFC. 14+.

Health Care Financing Administration. Sept. 2000. *Medicare & You 2001*. Publication No. HCFA-10050. Washington: U.S. Government Printing Office.

Health Care Financing Administration. March 2000. *Guide to Health Insurance for People with Medicare*. Publication N. HCFA-02110 Washington: U.S. Government Printing Office.

Jehle, Faustin F. July 1998. *The Complete and Easy Guide to Social Security, Healthcare Rights & Government Benefits*. Boca Raton: Emerson-Adams Press.

Social Security Administration. July 1999. *Social Security Supplemental Security Income*. SSA Publication No. 05-11000. Washington.

Social Security Administration. Sept. 1995. *Social Security Disability Programs Can Help*. SSA Publication No. 05-10057. Washington.

Social Security Administration. Aug. 2000. *Social Security Disability Benefits*. SSA Publication No. 05-10029. Washington.

U.S. Department of Labor Employment Standards Administration, Wage and Hour Division. Dec. 1996. Publication 1421. *Compliance Guide to the Family and Medical Leave Act*. Washington: U.S. Government Printing Office.

U.S. Department of Labor Employment Standards Administration, Wage and Hour Division. April 1995. WH Publication 1419. Federal Regulations Part 825. *The Family and Medical Leave Act of 1993*. Washington: U.S. Government Printing Office.

U.S. Department of Labor Employment Standards Administration, Wage and Hour Division. June 1993. WH Publication 1420. *Your Rights Under the Family and Medical Leave Act of 1993*. Washington: U.S. Government Printing Office.

U.S. Department of Labor Program. 1993. *The Family and Medical Leave Act of 1993*. Highlights Fact Sheet No. ESA 93-2. Washington: U.S. Government Printing Office.

U.S. Equal Employment Opportunity Commission, U.S. Department of Justice, Civil Rights Division. 1992. *The Americans with Disabilities Act, Questions and Answers*. Washington.

U.S. Equal Employment Opportunity Commission. 1991. *The Americans With Disabilities Act*. Washington.

United Network for Organ Sharing (UNOS). 1997. *What Every Patient Needs to Know.*

Chapter 8

Bonkovsky, H.L., B.F. Banner, A.L. Rothman. 1997. Iron and Chronic Viral Hepatitis. *Hepatology.* 25:759–767.

Brillanti S., F. Levantesi, L. Masi, M. Foli, L. Bolondi. 2000. Triple Antiviral Therapy as a New Option for Patients With Interferon Nonresponsive Chronic Hepatitis C. *Hepatology*. 32:630–634.

Causse, X., H. Godinot, M. Chevallier, P. Chossegros, F. Zoulim, D. Ouzan, J.P. Heyraud, T. Fontanes, J. Albrecht, C. Meschievitz, C. Trepo. 1991. Comparison of 1 or 3 MU of Interferon Alfa-2b and Placebo in Patients with Chronic Non-A, Non-B Hepatitis. *Gastroenterology.* 101:497–502.

Cheng, S.J., P.A.L. Bonis, J. Lau, N.Q. Pham, J.B. Wong. 2001. Interferon and Ribavirin for Patients with Chronic Hepatitis C Who Did Not Respond to Previous Interferon Therapy: A Meta-Analysis of Controlled and Uncontrolled Trials. *Hepatology.* 33:231–240.

Chemello, L., P. Bonetti, L. Cavallettoi, F. Talato, V. Donadon, P. Casarin, F. Belussi, M. Fezza, F. Noventa, P. Pontisso, L. Benvegnu, C. Casarin, A. Alberti, the TriVeneto Viral Hepatitis Group. 1995. Randomized Trial Comparing Three Different Regimens of Alpha-2a-Interferon in Chronic Hepatitis C. *Hepatology.* 22:700–706.

Davis, G.L., L.A. Balart, E.R. Schiff, K. Lindsay, H.C. Bodenheimer, R.P. Perrillo, W. Carey, I.M. Jacobson, J. Payne, J.L. Dienstag, D.H. Van Thiel, C. Tamburro, J. Lefkowitch, J. Albrecht, C. Meschievitz, T.J. Ortego, A. Gibas, and the Hepatitis Interventional Therapy Group. 1989. Treatment of Chronic Hepatitis C, with Recombinant Interferon Alfa. A Multicenter Randomized, Controlled Trial. *New England Journal of Medicine.* 321:1501–1506.

Davis, G.L., R. Esteban-Mur, V. Rustgi, J. Hoefs, S.C. Gordon, C. Trepo, M.L. Shiffman, S. Zeuzem, A. Craxi, M-H. Ling, J. Albrecht, for the International Hepatitis Interventional Therapy Group. 1998. Interferon Alfa-2b Alone Or In Combination With Ribavirin For The Treatment of Relapse of Chronic Hepatitis C. *New England Journal of Medicine.* 339:1493–9.

Di Bisceglie, A.M., P. Martin, C. Kassianides, M. Lisker-Melman, L. Murray, J. Waggoner, Z. Goodman, S.M. Banks, J. Hoofnagle. 1989. Recombinant Interferon Alfa Therapy for Chronic Hepatitis C. A Randomized, Double-blind, Placebo-controlled Trial. *New England Journal of Medicine.* 321:1506-1510.

Di Bisceglie, A.M., J. Thompson, N. Smith-Wilkaitis, E.M. Brunt, B.R. Bacon. 2001. Combination of Interferon and Ribavirin in Chronic Hepatitis C: Re-Treatment of Nonresponders to Interferon. *Hepatology.* 33:704-707.

Dusheiko, G.M., J.A. Roberts. 1995. Treatment of Chronic Type B and C Hepatitis with Interferon Alfa: an Economic Appraisal. *Hepatology.* 22:1863-1873.

Everson, G.T. 2000. Maintenance Interferon for Chronic Hepatitis C: More Issues than Answers? *Hepatology.* 32:436-438.

Hasan, F., L.J. Jeffers, M. DeMedina, K.R. Reddy, T. Parker, E.R. Schiff, M. Houghton, Q. Choo, G. Kuo. 1990. Hepatitis C-associated Hepatocellular Carcinoma. *Hepatology.* 12:589-591.

Hoofnagle, J.H., A.M. Di Bisceglie. 1997. The Treatment of Chronic Viral Hepatitis. New England Journal of Medicine. 336:347-356.

Hoofnagle, J.H., K.D. Mullen, D.B. Jones, V. Rustgi, A. Di Bisceglie, M. Peters, J.G. Waggoner, Y. Park, E.A. Jones. 1986. Treatment of Chronic Non-A, Non-B Hepatitis with Recombinant Human Alpha Interferon. *New England Journal of Medicine.* 315:1575-1578.

Koff, R.S., L.B. Seeff. 1995. Economic Modeling of Treatment in Chronic Hepatitis B and Chronic Hepatitis C: Promises and Limitations. *Hepatology.* 22:1880-82.

Lampertico, P., M. Rumi, R. Romeo, A. Craxi, R. Soffredini, D. Biassoni, M. Colombo. 1994. A Multicenter Randomized Controlled Trial of Recombinant Interferon-a2b in Patients with Acute Transfusion-associated Hepatitis C. *Hepatology.* 19:19-22.

Liang, T.J. 1998. Combination Therapy for Hepatitis C Infection. *New England Journal of Medicine.* 339:1549-50.

Lindsay, K.L., G.L. Davis, E.R. Schiff, H.C. Bodenheimer, L.A. Balart, J.L. Dienstag, R.P. Perrillo, C.H. Tamburro, J.S. Goff, G.T. Everson, M. Silva, W.N. Katkov, Z. Goodman, J.Y.N. Lau, G. Maertens, J. Gogate, B. Sanghvi, J. Albrecht, and the Hepatitis Interventional Therapy Group. 1996. Response to Higher Doses of Interferon Alfa-2b in Patients with Chronic Hepatitis C: A Randomised Multicenter Trial. *Hepatology.* 24:1034-1040.

Marcellin, P., N. Boyer, E. Giostra, C. Degott, A.M. Courouc, F. Degos, H. Coppere, P. Cales, P.K. Couzigou, J.P. Benhamou. 1991. Recombinant Human a-Interferon in Patients with Chronic Non-A, Non-B Hepatitis: a Multicenter Randomized Controlled Trial from France. *Hepatology.* 13:393-397.

Marcellin, P., M. Pouteau, M. Martinot-Peignoux, F. Degos, V. Duchatelle, N.M. Boyer, C. Lemonnier, C. Degott, S. Erlinger, P. Benhamou. 1995. Lack of Benefit of Escalating Dosage of Interferon Alfa in Patients with Chronic Hepatitis C. *Gastroenterology.* 109:156-165.

McHutchison, J.G., S.C. Gordon, E.R. Schiff, M.L. Shiffman, W.M. Lee, V.K. Rustgi, Z.D. Goodman, M-H. Ling, S. Cort, J. K. Albrecht, for the Hepatitis Interventional Therapy Group. 1998. Interferon Alfa-2b Alone Or In Combination With Ribavirin As Initial Treatment For Chronic Hepatitis C. *New England Journal of Medicine.* 339:1485-92.

Poynard, T., P. Bedossa, M. Chevallier, P. Mathurin, C. Lemonnier, C. Trepo, P. Couzigou, J.L Payen, M. Sajus, J.M. Costa, M. Vadaud, J.C. Chaput, the Multicenter Study Group. 1995. A Comparison of Three Interferon Alfa-2b Regimens for the Long-term Treatment of Chronic Non-A, Non-B Hepatitis. *New England Journal of Medicine.* 332:1457-62.

Poynard, T., V. Leroy, M. Cohard, T. Thevenot, P. Mathurin, P. Opolon, J.P. Zarski. 1996. Meta-Analysis of Interferon Randomized Trials in the Treatment of Viral Hepatitis C: Effects of Dose and Duration. *Hepatology.* 24:778-789.

Poynard, T., J. McHutchison, G.L. Davis, R. Esteban-Mur, Z. Goodman, P. Bedossa, J. Albrecht for the FIBROVIRC Project Group. 2000. Impact of Interferon Alfa-2b and Ribavirin on Progression of Liver Fibrosis in Patients with Chronic Hepatitis C. *Hepatology.* 32:1131-1137.

Reichard, O., H. Glaumann, A. Fryden, G. Norkrans, R. Schvarcz, A. Soonerborg, Z.B. Yun, O. Weiland. 1995. Two Year Biochemical, Virological, and Histological Follow-Up in Patients with Chronic Hepatitis C Responding in a Sustained Fashion to Interferon Alfa-2b Treatment. *Hepatology.* 21:918-922.

Serfaty, L., O. Chazouilleres, J.M. Pawlotsky, T. Andreani, C. Pellet, R. Poupon. 1996. Interferon Alfa Therapy in Patients with Chronic Hepatitis C and Persistently Normal Aminotransferase Activity. *Gastroenterology.* 5110:291-295.

Shiffman, M.L., C.M. Hofmann, V.A. Luketic, A.J. Sanyal, M.J. Contos, A.S. Mills. 1996. Improved Sustained Response Following Treatment of Chronic Hepatitis C by Gradual Reduction in the Interferon Dose. *Hepatology.* 24:21-26.

Shiffman, M.L., C.M. Hofmann, J. Gabbay, V.A. Luketic, R.K. Sterling, A. J. Sanyal, M.J. Contos, M.J. Ryan, C. Yoshida, V. Rustgi. 2000. Treatment of Chronic Hepatitis C in Patients Who Failed Interferon Monotherapy: Effects of Higher Doses of Interferon and Ribavirin Combination Therapy. *American Journal of Gastroenterology.* 95:2928-2935.

Simon, D.M., S.C. Gordon, M.M. Kaplan, R.S. Koff, F. Regenstein, G. Everson, Y.M. Lee, F. Weiner, A. Silverman, T. Plasse, D. Fedorczyk, M. Liao. 1997. Treatment of Chronic Hepatitis C with Interferon Alfa-n3: A Multicenter, Randomized, Open-Label Trial. *Hepatology.* 25:445-448.

Viladomiu, L., J. Genesca, J.I. Esteban, H. Allende, A. Gonzalez, J.C. Lopez-Talavera, R. Esteban, J. Guardia. 1992. Interferon-a in Acute Posttransfusion Hepatitis C: A Randomized, Controlled Trial. *Hepatology.* 15:767-769.

Woolf, G.M., L.M. Petrovic, S.E. Rojter, S. Wainwright, F.G. Villamil, W.N. Katkov, P. Michieletti, I.R. Wanless, F.R. Stermitz, J.J. Beck, J.M. Vierling. 1994. Acute Hepatitis Associated with the Chinese Herbal Product Jin Bu Huan. *Annals of Internal Medicine.* 121:729-735.

Chapter 9

Fried, M.W., M.L. Shiffman , R.K. Reddy, C. Smith, G. Marino, F. Goncales, D. Haeussinger, M. Diago, G. Carosi, J.P. Zarski, J. Hoffman, J. Yu. 2001. Pegylated (40 kDa) Interferon Alfa-2a in Combination with Ribavirin: Efficacy and Safety Results from a Phase III, Randomized, Actively-Controlled, Multicenter Study. *Gastroenterology.* 120 (suppl):A55.

Glue, P., R. Rouzier-Panis, C. Raffanel, R. Sabo, S.K. Gupta, M. Salfi, S. Jacobs, R.P. Clement, and the Hepatitis C Intervention Therapy Group. 2000. A Dose Ranging Study of Pegylated Interferon Alfa-2b and Ribavirin in Chronic Hepatitis C. *Hepatology* 32:647-653.

Heathcote, E.J., M.L. Shiffman, G.E. Cooksley, G.M. Dusheiko, S.S. Lee, L. Balart, R Reindollar, R.K. Reddy, T.L. Wright, A. Lin, J. Hoffman, J. De-Pamphilis. 2000. Peginterferon Alfa-2a in Patients with Chronic Hepatitis C and Cirrhosis. *New England Journal of Medicine.* 343:1673-1680.

Lindsay, K.L., C. Trepo, T. Hentges, M.L. Shiffman, S.C. Gordon, J.C. Hoefs, E.R. Schiff, Z.D. Goodman, M. Laughlin, R.Yao, J.K. Albrecht for the Hepatitis Interventional Therapy Group. 2001. A Randomized, Double-Blind Trial Comparing Pegylated Interferon Alfa-2b to Interferon Alfa-2b as Initial Treatment for Chronic Hepatitis C. *Hepatology.* 34:395-403.

Manns, M.P., J.G. McHutchison, S.C. Gordon, V.K. Rustgi, M. Shiffman, R. Reindollar, Z.D. Goodman, K. Koury, M-H. Ling, J.K. Albrecht and International Hepatitis Interventional Therapy Group. 2002. Peginterferon Alfa-2b Plus Ribavirin Compared with Interferon Alfa-2b Plus Rivavirin for Initial Treatment of Chronic Hepatitis C: A Randomised Trial. *The Lancet.* 358: 958-965.

Reddy, K.R., T.L. Wright, P.J. Pockros, M. Shiffman, G. Everson, R. Reindollar, M.W. Fried, P.P. Purdum, D. Jensen, C. Smith, W.M. Lee, T.D. Boyer, A. Lin, S. Pedder, J. DePamphilis. 2001. Efficacy and Safety of Pegylated (40 kD) Interferon alfa-2a Compared with Interferon alfa-2a in Noncirrhotic Patients with Chronic Hepatitis C. *Hepatology.* 33:433-438.

Shiffman, M.L. 2001. PEGylated Interferons: What Role Will They Play in the Treatment of Chronic Hepatitis C? *Current Gastroenterology Reports.* 3:30-37.

Sulkowski, M.S., R. Reindollar, J. Yu. 2000. Pegylated Interferon Alfa-2a (PE-GASYS) and Ribavirin Combination Therapy for Chronic Hepatitis C: A Phase II Open-Label Study. *Gastroenterology.* 188 (suppl 2):A950.

Zeuzem, S., S.V. Fienman, J. Rasenack, E.J. Heathcote, M-Y. Lai, E. Gane, J. O'-Grady, J. Reichen, M. Diago, A. Lin, J. Hoffman, M.J. Brunda. 2000. Peginterferon Alfa-2a in Patients with Chronic Hepatitis C. *New England Journal of Medicine.* 343:1666-1672.

Chapter 10

Burroughs, A.K. 2000. Posttransplantation Prevention and Treatment of Recurrent Hepatitis C. *Hepatology.* 6 (Suppl 2): S35-S40.

Chazouilleres, O., M. Kim, C. Combs, L. Ferrell, P. Bacchetti, J. Roberts, N.L. Ascher, P. Neuwald, J. Wilber, M. Urdea, S. Quan, R. Sanchez-Pescador, T.L. Wright. 1994. Quantitation of Hepatitis C Virus RNA in Liver Transplant Recipients. *Gastroenterology.* 106:994-999.

Dienstag, J.L. 1997. The Natural History of Chronic Hepatitis C and What We Should Do About It. *Gastroenterology.* 112:651-655.

Everhart, J.E., Y. Wei, H. Eng, M.R. Charlton, D.H. Persing, R.H. Weisner, J.J. Germer, J.R. Lake, R.K. Zetterman, J.H. Hoofnagle. 1999. Recurrent and New Hepatitis C Infection after Liver Transplantation. *Hepatology.* 29:1220-1226.

Everson, G.T., I. Kam. 1996. Liver Transplantation: Current Status and Unresolved Controversies. *Advances in Internal Medicine.* Vol. 42. London: Mosby-Year Book, Inc. pp. 505-553.

Everson, G.T., I. Kam. 2001. Immediate Postoperative Care. In *Transplantation of the Liver.* Editors Maddrey, W. C., E. R. Schiff, M. F. Sorrell. Lippincott Williams & Wilkins, Philadelphia. pp 131 – 162.

Fattovich, G., G. Giustina, F. Degos, F. Tremolada, G. Diodati, P. Almasio, F. Nevens, A. Solinas, D. Mura, J.T. Brouwer, H. Thomas, C. Njapoum, C. Casarin, P. Bonetti, P. Fuschi, J. Basho, A. Tocco, A. Bhalla, R. Galassini, F. Noventa, S.W. Schalm, G. Realdi. 1997. Morbidity and Mortality in Compensated Cirrhosis Type C: A Retrospective Follow-up Study of 384 Patients. *Gastroenterology.* 112:463-472.

Ferrell, L.D., T.L. Wright, J. Roberts, N. Ascher, J. Lake. 1992. Hepatitis C Viral Infection in Liver Transplant Recipients. *Hepatology.* 16:865-876.

Gane, E.J., N.V. Naoumov, K.P. Qian, M.U. Mondelli, G. Maertens, B.C. Portmann, J.Y.N. Lau, R. Williams. 1996. A Longitudinal Analysis of Hepatitis C Virus Replication Following Liver Transplantation. *Gastroenterology.* 110:167-177.

Gane, E.J., B.C. Portmann, N. Naoumov, H.M. Smith, J.A. Underhill, P.T. Donaldson, G. Maertens, R. Williams. 1996. Long-term Outcome of Hepatitis C Infection after Liver Transplantation. *New England Journal of Medicine.* 334:815-20.

Rosen, H.R. 2000. Retransplantation for Hepatitis C: Implications of Different Policies. *Hepatology.* 6 (Suppl 2):S41–S46.

Terrault, N.A. 2000. Hepatitis C and Liver Transplantation. *Seminars in Gastrointestinal Disease.* 11:96–114.

Testa, G., J.S. Crippin, G.J. Netto, R..M. Goldstein, L.W. Jennings, B.S. Brkic, B K. Brooks, M. F. Levy, T.A. Gonwa, G.B. Klintmalm. 2000. Liver Transplantation for Hepatitis C: Recurrence and Disease Progression in 300 Patients. *Liver Transplantation.* 6:553–561.

UNOS OPTN and Scientific Registry Data. From the Organ Procurement and Transplantation Network and the US Scientific Registry of Transplant Recipients, www.unos.org, July, 2001.

Chapter 11

Achkar, J-P., V. Araya, R.L. Baron, J.W. Marsh, I. Dvorchik, J. Rakela. 1998. Undetected Hepatocellular Carcinoma: Clinical Features and Outcome After Liver Transplantation. *Liver Transplantation and Surgery.* Vol. 4, No. 6 (Nov.):477–482.

Bruix, J. 1997. Treatment of Hepatocellular Carcinoma. *Hepatology.* 25:259–261.

Collier, J., M. Sherman. 1998. Screening for Hepatocellular Carcinoma. *Hepatology.* 27:273–278.

Di Bisceglie, Adrian M., R.L. Carithers, Jr., G.J. Gores. 1998. Hepatocellular Carcinoma. *Hepatology.* 28:1161–1165.

Di Bisceglie, A.M., S.E. Order, J.L. Klein, J.G. Waggoner, M.H. Sjogren, G. Kuo, M. Houghton, Q-L. Choo, J.H. Hoofnagle. 1991. The Role of Chronic Viral Hepatitis in Hepatocellular Carcinoma in the United States. *American Journal of Gastroenterology.* 86:335–338.

El-Serag, H.B., A.C. Mason. 1999. Rising Incidence of Hepatocellular Carcinoma in the United States. *New England Journal of Medicine.* 340:745–50.

Everson, G.T. 2000. Increasing Incidence and Pretransplantation Screening of Hepatocellular Carcinoma. *Liver Transplantation.* Vol. 6, No. 6, Suppl. 2 (Nov.):S2–S10.

Gordon, S.C., N. Bayati, A.L. Silverman. 1998. Clinical Outcome of Hepatitis C as a Function of Mode of Transmission. *Hepatology.* 28:562-567.

Imai, Yasuharu, S. Kawata, S. Tamura, I. Yabuuchi, S. Noda, M. Inada, Y. Maeda, Y. Shirai, T. Fukuzaki, I. Kaji, H. Ishikawa, Y. Matsuda, M. Nishikawa, K. Seki, Y. Matsuzawa. 1998. Relation of Interferon Therapy and Hepatocellular Carcinoma in Patients with Chronic Hepatitis C. *Annals of Internal Medicine.* 129:94-99.

Llovet, J.M., M. Sala, J. Bruix. 2000. Nonsurgical Treatment of Hepatocellular Carcinoma. *Hepatology.* 6 (Suppl 2):S11-S15.

Mazzaferro, V., E. Regalia, R. Doci, S. Andreola, A. Pulvirenti, F. Bozzetti, F. Montalto, M. Ammatuna, A. Morabito, L. Gennari. 1996. Liver Transplantation for the Treatment of Small Hepatocellular Carcinomas in Patients With Cirrhosis. *New England Journal of Medicine.* 334:693-699.

McMahon, B.J., T. London. 1991. Workshop on Screening for Hepatocellular Carcinoma. *Journal of the National Cancer Institute.* Vol. 83, No. 13 (July 3):916-919.

Penn, I. 1991. Hepatic Transplantation for Primary and Metastatic Cancers of the Liver. *Surgery.* 110:726-734.

Schalm, Solko W., G. Fattovich, J.T. Brouwer. 1997. Therapy of Hepatitis C: Patients With Cirrhosis. *Hepatology;* The National Institutes of Health Consensus Development Conference: Management of Hepatitis C. 26 (Suppl 1):128S-132S.

Serfaty, Lawrence, H. Aumaître, O. Chazouillères, A. Bonnand, O. Rosmorduc, R.E. Poupon, R. Poupon, 1998. Determinants of Outcome of Compensated Hepatitis C Virus-Related Cirrhosis. *Hepatology.* 27:1435-1440.

Takayama, T., M. Makuuchi, S. Hirohashi, M. Sakamoto, J. Yamamoto, K. Shimada, T. Kosuge, S. Okada, K. Takayasu, S. Yamasaki. 1998. Early Hepatocellular Carcinoma as an Entity with a High Rate of Surgical Cure. *Hepatology.* 28:1241-1246.

Wall, W.J., P.J. Marotta. 2000. Surgery and Transplantation for Hepatocellular Cancer. *Hepatology.* 6 (Suppl 2):S16-S22.

Williams, R., P. Rizzi. 1996. Treating Small Hepatocellular Carcinomas. *New England Journal of Medicine.* Vol. 334, No. 11:728-729.

Wong, L.L., W.M. Limm, R. Severino, L.M. Wong. 2000. Improved Survival with Screening for Hepatocellular Carcinoma. *Liver Transplantation.* Vol. 6, No. 3 (May):320-325.

World Health Organization. *Prevention of Liver Cancer.* Technical Report Series 691. Geneva: WHO, 1983.

Yuen, M-F, C-C. Cheng, I.J. Lauder, S-K. Lam, C. G-C. Ooi, C-L. Lai. 2000. Early Detection of Hepatocellular Carcinoma Increases the Chance of Treatment: Hong Kong Experience. *Hepatology.* 31:330-335.

Chapter 12

Abramowicz, M., Ed. 1995. Drugs for AIDS and Associated Infections. *The Medical Letter on Drugs and Therapeutics.* Vol. 37 (Issue 959):87-94.

"Basic Statistics-International Statistics." Jan. 2, 2001. *Centers for Disease Control & Prevention,* Divisions of HIV/AIDS Prevention. http://www.cdc.gov/hiv/stats/internat.htm. Nov. 2001.

Berger, A., M. v. Depka Prondzinski, H.W. Doerr, H. Rabenau, B. Weber. 1996. Hepatitis C Plasma Viral Load Is Associated With HCV Genotype But Not With HIV Coinfection. *Journal of Medical Virology.* 48:339-343.

Boyer, N., P. Marcellin, C. Degott, F. Degos, A. G. Saimot, S. Erlinger, J. P. Benhamou, and the Comite´ des Anti-Viraux. 1992. Recombinant Interferon-alpha for Chronic Hepatitis C in Patients Positive for Antibody to the Human Immunodeficiency Virus. *The Journal of Infectious Diseases.* 165:723-726.

Cacciola, I., T. Pollicino, G. Squadrito, G. Cerenzia, M.E. Orlando, G. Raimondo. 1999. Occult hepatitis B Virus Infection in Patients with Chronic Hepatitis Liver Disease. *New England Journal of Medicine.* 341:22-26.

Chang, C.J., Y.C. Ko, H.W. Liu. 2000. Serum Alanine Aminotransferase Levels in Relation to Hepatitis B and C Virus Infections among Drug Abusers in an Area Hyperendemic for Hepatitis B. *Digestive Disease and Science.* 45:1949-1952.

Chamot, E., B. Hirschel, J. Wintsch, C.F. Robert, V. Gabriel, J.J. Déglon, S. Yerly, L. Perrin. 1990. Loss of Antibodies Against Hepatitis C Virus in HIV-Seropositive Intravenous Drug Users. *AIDS.* 4:1275-1277.

Cribier, B., D. Rey, C. Schmitt, J.M. Lang, A. Kirn, F. Stoll-Keller . 1995. High Hepatitis C Viraemia and Impaired Antibody Response in Patients Coinfected with HIV. *AIDS.* 9, no. 10: 1131-1136.

Danner, S.A., A. Carr, J.M. Leonard, L.M. Lehman, F. Gudiol, J. Gonzales, A. Raventos, R. Rubio, E. Bouza, V. Pintado, A.G. Aguado, J.G. De Lomas, R. Delgado, J.C.C. Borleffs, A. Hsu, J. M. Valdes, C.A.B. Boucher, D.A. Cooper, for the European-Australian Collaborative Ritonavir Study Group. 1995. A Short-Term Study of the Safety, Pharmacokinetics, and Efficacy of Ritonavir, an Inhibitor of HIV-1 Protease. *New England Journal of Medicine.* 333:1528-33.

DenBrinker, M., F.W.N.M. Witt, P.M.E. Wertheim-VanDillen, S. Jurriaans, J. Weel, R. Van Leeuwen, N.G. Pakkor, P. Reiss, S.A. Danner, G.J. Weverling, J.M.A. Lange. 2000. Hepatitis B and C Virus Co-Infection and the Risk for Hepatotoxicity of Highly Active Anti-retroviral Therapy in HIV-1 Infection. *AIDS.* 14:2895-2902.

Dove, L.M., J. Alonzo, T.L. Wright. 2000. Clinicopathological Conference: Hepatitis C in a Patient with Human Immunodeficiency Virus Infection. *Hepatology.* 32:147-152.

Eyster, M.E., L.S. Diamondstone, J-M Lien, W.C. Ehmann, S. Quan, J.J. Goedert for the Multicenter Hemophilia Cohort Study. 1993. Natural History of Hepatitis C Virus Infection in Multitransfused Hemophiliacs Effect of Coinfection with HIV. *Journal of Acquired Immune Deficiency Syndrome.* 602-10.

Fong, T.L., A.M. DiBisceglie, J.G. Waggoner, S.M. Banks, J.H. Hoofnagle. 1991. The Significance of Antibody to Hepatitis C Virus in Patients with Chronic Hepatitis B. *Hepatology.* 14:64-67.

García-Samaniego, J., V. Soriano, J. Castilla, R. Bravo, A. Moreno, J. Carbó, A. Iñiguez, J. González, F. Muñoz, and The Hepatitis/HIV Spanish Study Group. 1997. Influence of Hepatitis C Virus Genotypes and HIV Infection on Histologic Severity of Chronic Hepatitis C. *The American Journal of Gastroenterology.* 92:7:1130-34.

Gostin, L.O., J.W. Ward, A.C. Baker. 1997. National HIV Case Reporting for the United States: A Defining Moment in the History of the Epidemic. *New England Journal of Medicine.* 337:1162-67.

Hayashi, P.H., N. Flynn, S.A. McCurdy, I..K. Kuramoto, P.V. Holland, J.B. Zeldis. 1991. Prevalence of Hepatitis C Virus Antibodies Among Patients Infected with Human Immunodeficiency Virus. *Journal of Medical Virology.* 33:177-80.

Kazemi-Shirazi, L., D. Petermann, C. Muller. 2000. Hepatitis B Virus DNA in Sera and Liver Tissue of HBsAg Negative Patients with Chronic Hepatitis C. *Journal of Hepatology.* 33:785-790.

Marriott, E., S. Navas, J. del Romero, S. Garcia, I. Castillo, J.A. Quiroga, V. Carreño. 1993. Treatment with Recombinant alpha-Interferon of Chronic Hepatitis C in Anti-HIV-Positive Patients. *Journal of Medical Virology.* 40:107-111.

Markowitz, M., M. Saag, W.G. Powderly, A.M. Hurley, A. Hsu, J.M. Valdes, D. Henry, F. Sattler, A. La Marca, J.M. Leonard, D.D. Ho. 1995. A Preliminary Study of Ritonavir, an Inhibitor of HIV-1 Protease, to Treat HIV-1 Infection. *New England Journal of Medicine.* 333:1534-9.

Pol, S., N. Trinh Thi, V. Thiers, F. Jaffredo, F. Camot, B. Lamorthe, H. Zylberberg, P. Bethelot, C. Bréchot, B. Nalpas. 1995. Chronic Hepatitis C of Drug Users: Influence of HIV Infection, Abstract No. 933. *Hepatology.* 22:340A.

Quan, C.M., M. Krajden, G.A. Grigoriew, I.R. Salit. 1993. Hepatitis C Virus Infection in Patients Infected with the Human Immunodeficiency Virus. *Clinical Infectious Diseases.* 17:117-9.

Ragni, M.V., O.K. Ndimbie, E.O. Rice, F.A. Bontempo, S. Nedjar. 1993. The Presence of Hepatitis C Virus HCV Antibody in Human Immunodeficiency Virus-Positive Hemophiliac Men Undergoing HCV "Seroreversion." *Blood.* 82:1010-15.

Remis, R.S., A. Dufour, M. Alary, J. Vincelette, J. Otis, B. Masse, B. Turmel, R. LeClerc, R. Parent, R. Lavoie. 2000. Association of Hepatitis B Virus Infection with Other Sexually Transmitted Infections in Homosexual Men. *American Journal of Public Health.* 90:1570-1574.

Rumi, M.G., M. Colombo, A. Gringeri, P.M. Mannucci. 1990. High Prevalence of Antibody to Hepatitis C Virus in Multitransfused Hemophiliacs with Normal Transaminase Levels. *Annals of Internal Medicine.* 112:379-380.

Sagnelli, E., N. Coppola, C. Scolastico, P. Filippini, T. Santantonio, T. Stroffolini, F. Piccinino. 2000. Virologic and Clinical Expressions of Reciprocal Inhibitory Effect of Hepatitis B, C, and Delta Viruses in Patients with Chronic Hepatitis. *Hepatology.* 32:1106-1110.

Selik, R.M., et al. April 2000. Increases In the Percentage with Liver Disease Among Deaths with HIV Infection. 10th International Symposium on Viral Hepatitis and Liver Disease; Atlanta, Georgia. (http://www.hivandhepatitis.com/hepb/bo4240002.html).

Sherman, K.E., S. Freeman, S. Harrison, L. Andron. 1991. Prevalence of Antibody to Hepatitis C Virus in Patients Infected with the Human Immunodeficiency Virus. *Journal of Infectious Diseases.* 163:414-415.

Soto, B., L. Rodrigo, J.A. del Olmo, M. Garcia-Begoechea, J. Hernandez-Quero, E. Lissen. 1994. Influence of Human Immunodeficiency Virus Type I Infection on the Natural History of Chronic Parenteral-Acquired Hepatitis C: A Multicenter Study on 547 Patients. Abstract No. 10. *Journal of Hepatology.* 21 S25.

Chapter 13

Alter, M. 1996. Epidemiology and Disease Burden of Hepatitis B and C. *Antiviral Therapy.* 1 (suppl 3): 9-14.

American Academy of Pediatrics, Committee on Infectious Diseases. 1998. Hepatitis C Virus Infection. *Pediatrics.* 101:481-485.

Bortolotti F., M. Resti, R. Giacchino, C. Azzari, N. Gussetti, C. Crivellaro, C. Barbera, F. Mannelli, L. Zancan, A. Bertolini. 1997. Hepatitis C Virus Infection and Related Liver Disease in Children of Mothers with Antibodies to the Virus. *Journal of Pediatrics.* 130:990-993.

Centers for Disease Control and Prevention. 1998. Recommendations for Prevention and Control of Hepatitis C Virus (HCV) Infection and HCV-Related Chronic Disease. *Morbidity and Mortality Weekly Report.* 47 (No. RR-19):22-25, 28-31.

Gibb, D.M., R.L. Goodall, D.T. Dunn, M. Healy, P. Neave, M. Cafferkey, K. Butler. 2000. Mother-to-Child Transmission of Hepatitis C Virus: Evidence for Preventable Peripartum Transmission. *Lancet.* 356:904-07.

Jonas, Maureen M. 1998. Viral Hepatitis. *Pediatric Gastrointestinal Disease,* Vol. II, 2nd Edition. Walker, W. A., P. R. Durie, J. R. Hamilton, J. A. Walker-Smith, J. B. Watkins, eds. St. Louis: Mosby. 1028-1041.

Kage, M., T. Fujisawa, K. Shiraki, T. Tanaka, T. Fujusawa, A. Kimura, K. Shimamatsu, E. Nakashima, M. Kojiro, M. Koike, Y. Tazawa, D. Abukawa, M. Okaniza, H. Takita, A. Matsui, T. Hayashi, T. Etou, S. Terawawa, K. Sugiyama, H. Tajiri, A. Yoden, Y. Kajiwara, M. Sata, Y. Uchimura, and the Child Liver Study Group of Japan. 1997. Pathology of Chronic Hepatitis C in Children. *Hepatology.* 26:771-775.

Zein, N. 1997. Vertical Transmission of Hepatitis C: To Screen or Not to Screen. *Journal of Pediatrics.* 130:859-861.

Chapter 14

Belli, L.S., C. Zavaglia, A.B. Alberti, F. Poli, G. Rondinara, E. Silini, E. Taioli, L. DeCarlis, M. Scalamogna, D. Forti, G. Pinzello, G. Ideo. 2000. Influence of Immunogenetic Background on the Outcome of Recurrent Hepatitis C after Liver Transplantation. Hepatology 31:1345-1350.

Bekkering, F.C., C. Stalgis, J.G. McHutchison, J.T. Brouwer, A.S. Perelson. 2001. Estimation of Early Hepatitis C Viral Clearance in Patients Receiving Daily Interferon and Ribavirin Therapy Using a Mathematical Model. *Hepatology.* 33:419-423.

Department of Health and Human Services, Food and Drug Administration. March 1990. From Test Tube to Patient: New Drug Development in the United States. *An FDA Consumer Special Report,* DHHS Publication No. 90-3168. Rockville: Jan. 1998, Rev.

Dulworth, Sherrie, S. Patel, B.S. Pyenson. 2000. "The Hepatitis Epidemic: Looking at the Tip of the Iceberg." New York: Milliman & Robertson, Inc.

Fanning, L.J., J. Levis, E. Kenny-Walsh, F. Wynne, M. Whelton, F. Shanahan. 2000. Viral Clearance in Hepatitis C (1b) Infection: Relationship with Human Leukocyte Antigen Class II in a Homogeneous Population. *Hepatology.* 31:1334-1337.

Grakoui, A., H.L. Hanson, C..M. Rice. 2001. Bad Time for Bonzo? Experimental Models of Hepatitis C Virus Infection, Replication, and Pathogenesis. *Hepatology.* 33:489-495.

Hepatitis Foundation International, "Walk on Washington – Mission Accomplished." *Hepatitis Alert.* Summer 2000:1.

Honda, M., S. Kaneko, H. Kawai, Y. Shirota, K. Kobayashi. 2001. Differential Gene Expression between Chronic Hepatitis B and C Hepatic Lesion. *Gastroenterology.* 120:955-966.

Howell, C., L. Jeffers, J.H. Hoofnagle. 2000. Hepatitis C in African Americans: Summary of a Workshop. *Gastroenterology.* 119:1385-1396.

Kim, W.R., J.B. Gross, J.J. Poterucha, G.R. Locke III, E.R. Dickson. 2001. Outcome of Hospital Care of Liver Disease Associated with Hepatitis C in the United States. *Hepatology.* 33:201-206.

Layden, J.E., T.J. Layden. 2001. How can Mathematics Help Us Understand HCV? *Gastroenterology.* 120:1546-1549.

Lee, P.A., L. M. Blatt, K. S. Blanchard, K. S. Bouhana, P.A. Pavco, L. Bellon, J.A. Sandberg. 2000. Pharmacokinetics and Tissue Distribution of a Ribozyme Directed Against Hepatitis C Virus RNA Following Subcutaneous or Intravenous Administration in Mice. *Hepatology.* 32:640-646.

McHutchison, J.G., T. Poynard, S. Pianko, S.C. Gordon, A.E. Reid, J. Dienstag, T. Morgan, R. Yao, J. Albrecht, for the International Hepatitis Interventional Therapy Group (HIT). 2000. The Impact of Interferon Plus Ribavirin on Response to Therapy in Black Patients with Chronic Hepatitis C. *Gastroenterology.* 119:1317-1323.

Orland, J.R., T.L. Wright, S. Cooper. 2001. Acute Hepatitis C. *Hepatology.* 33:321-327.

Pawlotsky, J.-M. 2000. Hepatitis C Virus Resistance to Antiviral Therapy. *Hepatology.* 32:889-896.

Sakamoto, N., C.H. Wu, G.Y. Wu. 1996. Intracellular Cleavage of Hepatitis C Virus RNA and Inhibition of Viral Protein Translation by Hammerhead Ribozymes. *Journal of Clinical Investigation.* 98:2720-8.

Sarnow, P. 1995. *Current Topics in Microbiology and Immunology.* Volume 203; Berlin Heidelberg: Springer-Verlag. pp: 99–112.

Sherman, K.E., M. Sjogren, R.L. Creager, M.A. Damiano, S. Freeman, S. Lewey, D. Davis, S. Root, F.L. Weber, K.G. Ishak, Z.D. Goodman. 1998. Combination Therapy With Thymosin a1 and Interferon for the Treatment of Chronic Hepatitis C Infection: A Randomized, Placebo-Controlled Double-Blind Trial. *Hepatology.* 27:1128–1135.

Taylor, D.R. Hepatitis C Virus and Interferon Resistance: It's More Than Just PKR. 2001. *Hepatology.* 33:1547–1549.

Wu, C.H., G.Y. Wu. 1998. Targeted Inhibition of Hepatitis C Virus-Directed Gene Expression in Human Hepatoma Cell Lines. *Gastroenterology.* 114:1304–1312.

Zeuzem, S., E. Herrmann, J-H Lee, J. Fricke, A.U. Neumann, M. Modi, G. Colucci, W.K. Roth. 2001. Viral Kinetics in Patients with Chronic Hepatitis C Treated with Standard or Peginterferon alfa-2a. *Gastroenterology.* 120:1438–1447.

Index

LIVING WITH HEPATITIS B
A Survivor's Guide
THIRD REVISED EDITION
by Gregory T. Everson, M.D., F.A.C.P., and Hedy Weinberg

"I am grateful that this book was written. It is unique and fills an important niche."
—From the foreword by Steve Bingham
Co-owner, *Hepatitis B Information and Support List*

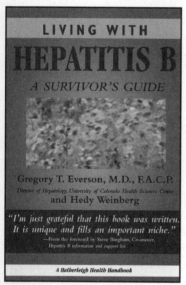

ISBN 1-57826-084-1
$15.95

Chronic hepatitis B currently affects almost 1.25 million Americans and can lead to cirrhosis, liver cancer, and the need for liver transplantation.

Now, the team that wrote the best-selling *Living With Hepatitis C* offers hepatitis B sufferers the same authoritative information, expert answers, practical guidance, hope, and inspiration. In *Living With Hepatitis B: A Survivor's Guide,* noted hepatologist Gregory T. Everson, M.D., F.A.C.P. and writer and hepatitis patient Hedy Weinberg offer a wide range of vital information that will allow you to make informed choices about your health, your treatment, and your finances.

Topics include:

* The safety and effectiveness of the HBV vaccine
* How to avoid infecting others
* How to understand blood tests and biopsies
* Nutrition tips for a healthier liver
* Treatment options and research trends
* Cutting medical costs

Written especially for patients and their families, *Living With Hepatitis B* presents an extremely complex and emotionally challenging subject in understandable language with an optimistic tone. It is necessary reading for anyone affected by hepatitis B.

THE SECRET STRENGTH OF DEPRESSION

by Frederic Flach, M.D.

"Turn depression into expression—and gain new energy zest, and self-respect…"
—*The Denver Post*

"…can make you feel better just by reading it."
—*The Boston Globe*

"Informed, hopeful and helpful look at the malaise in layman's terms… Dr Flach's credentials lend weight to his views and insights."
—*Publishers Weekly*

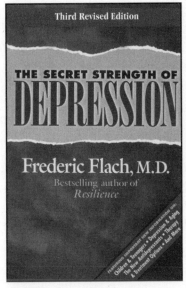

ISBN 1-57826-114-7
$15.95

The Secret Strength of Depression, first published in 1974, has long been acclaimed as one of the clearest and most helpful books on the subject of depression.

Fully revised and updated for the new millennium, this new paperback edition includes the latest discoveries in the treatment of depression. It has been expanded to include reports of the myths and miracles of the new antidepressants, the most recent findings on the biology of depression in women, and new information on depression in adolescents and the elderly.

In these uncertain times, more and more Americans are struggling with feelings of depression and anxiety. According to Dr. Flach, depression is a natural, healthy reaction to stressful events or major lifestyle changes such as marriage, divorce, career changes, or retirement. By acknowledging that depression can be an adaptive response to certain situations, Dr. Flach helps readers to tap their creative energies to turn depression into a positive force for personal growth.

WOMEN AND ANXIETY
A Step-by-Step Program for Managing Anxiety and Depression
REVISED EDITION
by Helen A. DeRosis, M.D.

Anxiety and Depression Are Facts of Life, but You Don't Have to Live with Them!

"A book every woman—married, single, working, or home-oriented—could use to help her live a fuller, free-of-fear life"
—*Ladies Home Journal*

"...a timely, well-written guide that ought to go a long way in helping today's women cope with the stresses of modern life."
—*San Francisco Sunday Examiner & Chronicle*

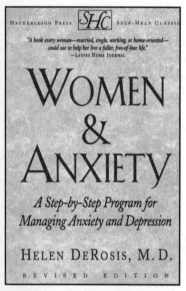

ISBN 1-886330-99-9
$14.95

Single parenthood. Marriage problems. AIDS. Sexual freedom. Divorce. Career demands. The glass ceiling. Run with the Wolves or play by The Rules. Pro-Life. Choice. Alternative lifestyles.

No wonder women are anxious and depressed. Never before have women been confronted with so many bewildering choices and so many incessant demands. How do women cope? How can they defeat self-defeating attitudes and actions? How can they conquer their fears, win the battle with anxiety and triumph over depression?

Women and Anxiety, first published in 1979, has been hailed as a book that "every woman—married, single, working, or home-oriented—could use to help her live a fuller, free-of-fear life." Now completely revised and updated, *Women and Anxiety* offers readers a new, dynamic, and easy step-by-step program. With sensible suggestions and solutions, this book will show you how to turn anxiety into a positive force in your life and how to learn to channel it in healthy and constructive ways.

RESILIENCE

How to Bounce Back When the Going Gets Tough!
by Frederic Flach, M.D.

"Part practical and part inspirational...Written with clarity...contains short, readable examples for all aspects of life...useful to laypersons in times of crisis."
—*The New England Journal of Medicine*

There's no escaping stress. It appears on our doorstep uninvited in the shattering forms of death and divorce, or even in the pleasant experiences of promotion, marriage, or a long-held wish fulfilled. Anything that upsets the delicate balance of our daily lives creates stress. So why do some people come out of a crisis feeling better than ever, while others never seem quite themselves again?

Drawing on thirty years of case studies from his own psychiatric practice, Dr. Flach reveals the remarkable antidote to the destructive qualities of stress: RESILIENCE.

ISBN 1-886330-95-6
$14.95

Readers will discover:

- How to develop the 14 traits that will make you more resilient
- Why "falling apart" is the smartest step to take on the road to resilence
- How to break down your body's resilience blockers and gain strength
- The sanity-saving technique of distracting yourself
- The helpful five-step plan for creative problem solving
- How developing your self-worth and your own unique gifts leads to resilience
- The power of language to destroy and to heal
- How to redefine your problem and restructure your pain to create a life you can handle, a life you can learn from and enjoy!